The Organic Diet Adventure

Learn the Secrets to Long-Term Health, Weight Loss, and Proper Nutrition

Elmer Gordon

Dedication

Dedicated to all those seeking vigorous health, mindful living, and a greener future. May your experience with '**The Organic Diet Adventure**' be inspiring, empowering, and transformative. Here's to growing sustenance for the body, mind, and earth, one organic decision at a time.

Table of Contents

Acknowledgement

I would like to express our deepest appreciation to everyone who helped create "The Organic Diet Adventure." Special thanks researchers, editors, and designers who worked tirelessly to bring this book to life. I also want to thank the farmers, producers, and supporters of organic agriculture whose enthusiasm and dedication inspire us every day. Finally, I want to thank our readers for joining me on this path to a better lifestyle and a more sustainable future. Your encouragement and excitement boost our efforts to raise awareness about the advantages of an organic diet.

Introduction

Growing Interest in Organic Diets

In recent years, interest in organic foods has grown tremendously. What was previously seen as a niche dietary option has now become a mainstream phenomenon, attracting the attention of health-conscious consumers, environmental campaigners, and even food business titans. The organic movement is more than simply a fleeting fad; it signifies a significant change in consumer behavior and attitudes.

Organic diets appeal to people because they offer purity and sustainability. Organic agriculture promotes natural and ecologically friendly approaches over conventional agricultural methods, which mainly depend on industrial pesticides, fertilizers, and genetically modified organisms (GMOs). This dedication to protecting land integrity and encouraging biodiversity speaks to a rising portion of the people concerned about our planet's health.

Furthermore, growing awareness of the possible health concerns connected with synthetic chemical exposure has increased the demand for organic foods. Consumers are more suspicious of pesticide-laden items and prefer organically farmed-food and pasture-raised meats. The aim to reduce one's exposure to pollutants and increase general well-being has propelled the organic food movement.

Beyond environmental and health concerns, organic diets are appealing because they offer higher flavor and nutritional value. Organic food advocates emphasize the superior tastes and textures of organically cultivated fruits and vegetables, as well as their greater quantities of vitamins, minerals, and antioxidants. Organic diets provide a means for people to reconnect with nature while also savoring the real essence of fresh, healthful products.

The Importance of Good Nutrition for Long-Term Health and Weight Management

Proper nutrition is the foundation of long-term health and weight control. The food we consume not only gives our bodies the fuel they need to operate, but it also helps to avoid chronic illnesses, maintain a healthy weight, and promote general well-being. However, in today's fast-paced world of processed meals and fad diets, many people need help to eat a healthy diet.

The repercussions of insufficient nutrition are far-reaching and severe. Inadequate nutritional intake may impair the immune system, raise the risk of cardiovascular disease, and lead to obesity and other metabolic diseases. A diet high in whole foods, fruits, vegetables, lean proteins, and healthy fats, on the other hand, may boost immunity, promote peak energy, and improve mental clarity and attention.

Weight control is another important part of a good diet. Obesity has reached epidemic proportions globally, causing a slew of health issues such as diabetes, hypertension, and stroke. While crash diets and restricted eating programs may provide temporary effects, they often fail to generate long-term weight reduction or enhance general health. Instead, a balanced and nutrient-dense diet, along with frequent physical exercise, is critical for obtaining and maintaining a healthy weight over time.

Furthermore, healthy nutrition is concerned with both the amount and the quality of the food we eat. Choosing nutrient-dense meals versus processed and refined options may have a substantial impact on our health results. By focusing on complete, organic foods that are devoid of synthetic chemicals and additives, we can provide our bodies with the nutrition they need to survive and develop.

An Overview of the Organic Diet Adventure

The organic diet experience is about exploration, discovery, and change. It's a journey into the world of healthy foods, bright tastes, and sustainable living. At its foundation, the organic diet journey is about adopting a holistic approach to eating that feeds the body, mind, and spirit.

Throughout this voyage, readers will discover the secrets of long-term health, weight reduction, and good nutrition. They'll learn how to confidently navigate the grocery store aisles, picking the freshest organic food and ethically produced meat. They will know the pleasures of preparing simple but tasty meals with fresh ingredients and inventive recipes.

The organic diet experience, however, is more than simply what we consume; it is also about how we eat and live. It is about developing a better respect for the food we eat and its effects on our bodies and the environment. It's about creating a stronger connection to the natural world and understanding our duty as planet stewards.

As readers begin on this journey, they will be led by professional counsel, practical recommendations, and inspirational anecdotes from real-life people who have seen the transformational power of organic eating. Whether they want to improve their health, reduce weight, or adopt a more sustainable lifestyle, the organic diet experience has something for everyone.

In the following chapters, we will explore the concepts of organic diets, investigate the science behind organic nutrition, and uncover delectable dishes that highlight the wealth of tastes and nutrients found in organic foods. We will also discuss frequent problems and misunderstandings about organic eating and provide practical solutions to overcome them.

So, come along on this fascinating and life-changing journey as we discover the keys to long-term health, weight reduction, and adequate nutrition using the power of organically cultivated foods. Together, we will begin a journey toward a healthier, happier, and more vibrant way of life.

Chapter 1

Definition and Principles of the Organic Diet

In the midst of dietary advice and nutritional trends, the phrase "organic diet" has developed as a symbol of health and sustainability. But what precisely does it mean to follow an organic diet, and what principles guide this way of eating? In this chapter, we'll look at the organic diet's origins, standards, and guiding beliefs.

Understanding The Organic Diet

The organic diet is a nutritional strategy that focuses on eating foods cultivated or produced without synthetic pesticides, fertilizers, hormones, or genetically modified organisms (GMOs). These foods are grown utilizing organic agricultural practices that promote soil health, biodiversity, and ecological balance. The word "organic" refers to a set of farming methods and standards developed by regulatory authorities such as the United States

Department of Agriculture (USDA) and the European Union. These standards specify the techniques and chemicals that may be used in the manufacturing, processing, and labeling of organic foods, providing transparency and integrity across the supply chain. In practical terms, organic foods include fruits, vegetables, grains, meats, dairy products, and processed meals manufactured with organic components. By selecting organic, customers may decrease their exposure to potentially dangerous chemicals while also supporting ecologically friendly agricultural techniques.

The organic diet is based on a set of key concepts that represent a comprehensive approach to food and nutrition. These principles provide an emphasis not just on food quality but also on human health, environmental sustainability, and social justice. Some of the main elements of the organic diet are:

- Health and Nutrition: Organic foods are regarded for their greater nutritional value, with higher amounts of vitamins, minerals, antioxidants, and phytonutrients than conventionally cultivated rivals. Prioritizing organic foods may help people improve their general health and wellbeing while also lowering their risk of chronic illnesses, including obesity, diabetes, and cardiovascular disease.
- Environmental Sustainability: Organic agricultural techniques aim to reduce environmental impact by

protecting soil health, conserving water resources, and fostering biodiversity. Crop rotation, cover cropping, and natural pest management are among the strategies used by organic farmers to improve soil fertility and minimize dependency on synthetic fertilizers. By purchasing organic, customers may support agricultural systems that promote ecological care while mitigating the harmful consequences of industrial agriculture on the environment.

- Animal Welfare: In addition to plant-based meals, the organic diet includes animal products farmed under rigorous animal welfare guidelines. Organic cattle have access to outdoor grass and are reared without the use of antibiotics or growth hormones. By purchasing organic meat, dairy, and eggs, people can promote animal welfare and guarantee that their food choices are consistent with their ethical views.
- Social Responsibility: The organic diet is founded on values of social justice and fairness, emphasizing the value of ethical labor practices, community participation, and economic development. Organic farming creates opportunities for small-scale farmers and rural communities by encouraging local food systems and connecting producers and consumers. Individuals who support organic

agriculture may create a more fair and equitable food system for all stakeholders.

Origins and Evolution of the Organic Diet.

The organic diet may be traced back to the early twentieth century when pioneering farmers and philosophers started to criticize agriculture's industrialization, dependence on synthetic chemicals, and monoculture farming. Visionaries, including Sir Albert Howard, Rudolf Steiner, and J.I. Rodale, pushed for holistic farming practices that prioritize soil health, biodiversity, and sustainability. The organic movement gained traction in the 1960s and 1970s, fueled by worries about industrial agriculture's environmental impact, the health impacts of chemical pesticides and fertilizers, and the decline of rural communities. Grassroots groups, such as the Soil Association in the United Kingdom and the Organic Farming Research Foundation in the United States, were crucial in promoting organic farming techniques and fighting for government assistance.

In response to rising consumer demand for organic foods, governments throughout the globe established regulatory frameworks to define and certify organic goods. In the United States, the Organic Foods Production Act (OFPA) was enacted in 1990, establishing the framework for the USDA National Organic

Program (NOP) and the establishment of national organic standards. The USDA organic certification program establishes severe norms for organic farming, processing, and labeling, assuring that goods wearing the USDA organic stamp satisfy rigorous organic production standards. Organic certification is administered by qualified certifying agencies that audit farms and food processors to ensure they meet organic requirements. In addition to government laws, third-party organizations like as the Organic Trade Association (OTA) and the Non-GMO Project provide certification and labeling systems to assist customers in identifying organic and non-GMO goods in the marketplace. These certification systems act as a reliable emblem of honesty and integrity, allowing customers to make educated decisions about the foods they consume.

Key Components of an Organic Diet

Fruits and vegetables are the cornerstone of an organic diet, supplying critical vitamins, minerals, and antioxidants that promote general health and wellbeing. Organic produce is farmed without synthetic pesticides, herbicides, or fertilizers, avoiding exposure to potentially dangerous chemicals while maintaining nutritional integrity. Crop rotation, composting, and biological pest management are examples of organic farming methods that contribute to soil fertility and biodiversity, resulting in healthier plants and higher-quality products. Organic fruits and vegetables are also less likely to have pesticide residues, making them a more nutritious option for customers, particularly pregnant women, children, and those with impaired immune systems.

Whole grains and legumes are essential components of the organic diet, offering a wealth of complex carbs, fiber, and proteins. Organic grains, including wheat, rice, oats, and quinoa, are grown without synthetic fertilizers or genetically modified seeds, retaining their original nutritional profile and taste. Similarly, organic legumes like beans, lentils, and chickpeas are farmed using sustainable farming techniques that improve soil health and decrease environmental impact. These plant-based protein sources are not only healthful but also adaptable, serving as the foundation for a variety of savory recipes, including soups, stews, salads, and casseroles.

Organic meat and dairy products are made from animals bred in compliance with rigorous animal welfare guidelines and organic agricultural techniques. Organic cattle have access to outdoor pasture and are fed organic feed that does not include synthetic hormones, antibiotics, or genetically engineered components. Organic meat, poultry, eggs, and dairy products allow customers to promote animal welfare while also reducing their exposure to antibiotics and other toxic substances used in conventional animal husbandry. Organic meat and dairy are also richer in essential elements like omega-3 fatty acids and conjugated linoleic acid (CLA), making them a better option for anyone looking to improve their nutritional intake.

In addition to fresh foods, the organic diet includes a range of processed items containing organic components. These include packaged snacks, cereals, breads, drinks, and frozen dinners made using organic farming processes and certified organic components. While processed organic foods may have additional sugars, fats, and preservatives, they are often devoid of synthetic chemicals and genetically engineered substances present in conventional processed meals. As with any food item, it's important to read labels carefully and choose organic processed foods that correspond to your dietary choices and nutritional objectives.

Advantages of Selecting Organic Foods

In a world where food options are many and health concerns are crucial, the decision to eat organic foods stands out as a symbol of wellbeing and sustainability. In this chapter, we will look at the many advantages of eating organic foods, including their better nutritional profile, favorable influence on human health, environmental sustainability, and social responsibility.

Superior nutrition profile

One key advantage of consuming organic foods is their increased nutritional value. Organic fruits, vegetables, cereals, and dairy products are often higher in critical vitamins, minerals, antioxidants, and phytonutrients than conventionally cultivated competitors.

Higher antioxidant content: Studies have shown that organic fruits and vegetables contain more antioxidants, including vitamin C, vitamin E, and polyphenols. Antioxidants are essential for protecting cells from oxidative damage, decreasing inflammation, and lowering the risk of chronic illnesses, including heart disease, cancer, and neurological disorders.

More nutrient-dense: Organic foods are also more nutrient-dense, which means they have greater concentrations of vital elements in each serving. For example, organic fruit has been discovered to include greater quantities of vitamins and minerals such as vitamin A, vitamin C, calcium, magnesium, and iron, all of which are essential for general health and wellbeing.

Balanced fatty acid profile: Organic meat and dairy products provide more beneficial elements, such as omega-3 fatty acids and conjugated linoleic acid (CLA), which have been linked to better cardiovascular, cognitive, and immunological performance. By selecting organic meat and dairy, customers may ensure a more balanced fatty acid profile and lower their risk of chronic illnesses related to unbalanced fat consumption.

Reduced exposure to harmful chemicals

One key reason for selecting organic foods is to limit exposure to potentially dangerous chemicals used in conventional agriculture. Organic farming techniques limit the use of synthetic pesticides, herbicides, fertilizers, and genetically modified organisms (GMOs), reducing the possibility of chemical contamination in food and the environment.

Pesticide residue-free: Organic fruits and vegetables are cultivated without the use of synthetic pesticides, which lowers the danger of pesticide residues on the product's surface. Organic food has much lower amounts of pesticide residues than conventionally produced produce, making it a safer option for consumers, particularly pregnant women, children, and those with impaired immune systems.

Hormone-Free: Organic meat and dairy products are derived from animals reared without the use of synthetic hormones, antibiotics, or growth boosters. Conventional animal husbandry often uses antibiotics and hormones to promote development and prevent sickness, raising worries about antibiotic resistance and hormone disruption in humans.

Non-GMO: Organic foods are also devoid of genetically modified organisms (GMOs), which are creatures with genetic material that has been purposefully altered in a laboratory. GMOs are widely employed in traditional agriculture to boost crop yields, improve pest and disease resistance, and increase herbicide tolerance.

Differentiating Organic and Conventional Foods

In an age of many food options, the difference between organic and conventional foods has become more significant for consumers looking to make educated diet and lifestyle decisions. In this chapter, we will look at the fundamental distinctions between organic and conventional foods, including production techniques, labeling standards, and possible effects on human health, environmental sustainability, and social responsibility.

Understanding organic foods

Production methods: Organic foods are grown using agricultural practices that promote soil health, biodiversity, and ecological balance, with little use of synthetic chemicals, pesticides, fertilizers, and genetically modified organisms (GMOs). Organic farmers use a range of sustainable strategies, such as crop rotation, cover cropping, composting, and natural pest management, to improve soil fertility and plant health without depending on chemicals.

Certification requirements: Foods that are labeled and marketed as organic must fulfill high criteria and certification requirements set by regulatory agencies such as the United States Department of Agriculture (USDA) or the European Union. These standards specify the techniques and chemicals that may be used in the manufacturing, processing, and labeling of organic foods, providing transparency and integrity across the supply chain.

Labeling: Organic foods are marked with the USDA organic logo or other certified organic labels to show that they were grown and processed in accordance with organic guidelines. The USDA organic mark falls into three categories:

- "100% Organic": Products with this mark include solely organic components and are manufactured and processed without the use of synthetic chemicals or additions.
- "Organic": Products branded "organic" include at least 95% organic components, with the remaining 5% made up of authorized non-organic substances that are not accessible in organic form.
- "Made with Organic Ingredients": Products branded as "made with organic ingredients" include at least 70% organic components, with the remaining 30% made up of authorized non-organic ingredients.

Understanding conventional foods

Production methods: Conventional foods are grown using traditional agricultural practices that depend extensively on synthetic chemicals, pesticides, fertilizers, and genetically modified organisms (GMOs) to increase crop yields and manage pests and illnesses. Monoculture farming, in which large-scale single-crop plants are grown across vast areas, is common among conventional farmers, and it often results in soil deterioration, erosion, and biodiversity loss.

Regulations and Labeling: Government organizations such as the Food and Drug Administration (FDA) and the Environmental Protection Agency (EPA) regulate conventional foods by establishing rules and safety requirements for their manufacture and processing. Traditional foods, unlike organic foods, are not obliged to fulfill stringent certification or labeling regulations regarding agricultural techniques or ingredient origin.

Pesticide use: One significant distinction between organic and conventional foods is the usage of synthetic pesticides and chemicals. Conventional farming mainly depends on the use of synthetic pesticides, herbicides, and fertilizers to manage pests, weeds, and illnesses, which often leave chemical residues on food items and pose health hazards to consumers.

Key Differences between Organic and Conventional Foods

Production methods: Organic foods are grown using sustainable agricultural techniques that promote soil health, biodiversity, and ecological balance while limiting the use of synthetic chemicals and pesticides. Conventional foods are produced using traditional farming practices that depend extensively on synthetic chemicals, pesticides, and fertilizers to increase crop yields while controlling pests and illnesses.

Certification and labelling: Organic foods are subject to stringent certification and labeling regulations set by regulatory agencies such as the USDA. Items have the USDA organic logo or other certified organic labels. Conventional foods are not obliged to fulfill strict certification or labeling criteria pertaining to agricultural techniques or ingredient origin.

Pesticide residues: Organic foods are less likely to have pesticide residues than conventional foods since organic farming restricts the use of synthetic pesticides and chemicals. Conventional foods may include pesticide residues from the use of synthetic pesticides and chemicals in standard agricultural techniques, which might pose health hazards to consumers.

Benefits of Choosing Organic Food

Health and Nutrition: When compared to conventionally farmed meals, organic foods frequently include more critical elements such as vitamins, minerals, antioxidants, and phytonutrients. Organic foods have no synthetic pesticides, herbicides, or fertilizers, lowering exposure to potentially dangerous chemicals and increasing general health and wellbeing.

Finally, the organic diet develops as a holistic approach to food consumption that incorporates nutritional and moral concerns. The organic movement has grown into a worldwide phenomenon backed by stringent regulatory frameworks and certification requirements. Its concentration on foods grown without synthetic pesticides, fertilizers, or GMOs provides greater nutrition while simultaneously reducing exposure to hazardous chemicals. Furthermore, organic farming techniques improve soil health, biodiversity, and animal welfare, thus contributing to environmental sustainability and social responsibility. Understanding the differences between organic and conventional foods enables consumers to make informed decisions, resulting in a healthier, more sustainable food system that promotes individual and societal wellbeing. Thus, the organic diet is more than simply a nutritional preference; it is a whole lifestyle choice with far-reaching consequences for health, society, and the environment.

As we move forward, the next chapter offers a new perspective on the relationship between nutrition, health, and the environment. It will emphasize the value of organic foods, which are grown with consideration for both our health and the environment. We'll learn how organic meals may build a foundation for our future wellbeing using simple yet strong ideas. We'll also look at how organic foods help to avoid sickness, support weight control, and nurture a better world. We'll look at how nutrient-dense, pesticide-free foods help both our health and the environment. Despite problems like accessibility and cost, the future seems promising. Organic foods may become more accessible and cheaper for everyone as awareness grows and collaborative action is taken. We'll go on a journey to a better, healthier future, one mouthful at a time.

Chapter 2

The Effect of Diet on Overall Health.

Diet appears as a vital thread tying together the fabric of human health. The foods we eat significantly impact our physical, mental, and emotional health, affecting everything from energy levels and immune function to mood control and illness risk. In this chapter, we will examine the substantial influence of food on general health, diving into the complex interactions between nutrition, metabolism, and physiological function.

Foundation of Health:

At its heart, a healthy diet is high in nutrients such as antioxidants, vitamins, minerals, and plant-based nutrients, which support optimum physiological function and promote overall health. Nutrient-dense diets act as building blocks for cellular repair and regeneration, powering metabolic processes and strengthening immunological defenses against infection and illness.

A healthy diet contains vital nutrients as well as a balanced ratio of macronutrients (carbohydrates, proteins, and fats) that supply energy and promote cellular activity. Carbohydrates are the body's and brain's principal fuel sources, while proteins are required for tissue repair and muscle development. Fats are necessary for hormone synthesis and nutrition absorption.

Water is another essential component of a healthy diet since it transports nutrients throughout the body, eliminates waste, and regulates metabolic processes. Adequate hydration is critical for maintaining cellular hydration, sustaining cognitive function, and improving athletic performance.

The Role of Diet in Disease Prevention

Numerous studies have shown that nutrition has a significant influence on cardiovascular health, with diets high in fruits, vegetables, whole grains, and lean meats linked with a lower risk of heart disease, stroke, and hypertension. In contrast, diets heavy in saturated fat, cholesterol, and processed foods have been related to an increased risk of cardiovascular disease and metabolic disorders.

Diet plays an important role in controlling metabolism and blood sugar levels. Dietary patterns that support stable blood glucose management are linked to a lower risk of type 2 diabetes and insulin resistance. Foods abundant in fiber, such as fruits, vegetables, and whole grains, help decrease sugar absorption into the circulation, while lean proteins and healthy fats enhance satiety and insulin sensitivity.

The immune system requires a consistent supply of critical nutrients; shortages in crucial vitamins and minerals decrease immunological responses and increase vulnerability to infection and illness. Diets high in immune-boosting foods, including vitamin C, vitamin D, zinc, and antioxidants, may strengthen immunological defenses, decrease inflammation, and increase pathogen resistance.

Gastrointestinal health

The gut microbiome, a complex ecology of bacteria, fungi, and other microorganisms that live in the gastrointestinal tract, is crucial for digestion, nutritional absorption, and immunological function. Diet has a significant impact on the composition and diversity of the gut microbiome, with fiber-rich, fermented, and prebiotic-rich foods helping to maintain a healthy balance of beneficial gut bacteria and lowering the risk of gastrointestinal disorders like irritable bowel syndrome (IBS) and inflammatory bowel disease (IBD).

The Effect of Diet on Mental Health

The brain is very sensitive to dietary influences, with some nutrients having important roles in cognitive performance, mood control, and mental health. Omega-3 fatty acids, found in fatty fish, flaxseeds, and walnuts, promote brain health and neurotransmitter function, while antioxidants like vitamin E and flavonoids protect against oxidative stress and cognitive decline.

Dietary patterns have been connected to mood regulation and mental health outcomes, with diets high in fruits, vegetables, whole grains, and omega-3 fatty acids being associated with lower rates of depression, anxiety, and mood disorders. In contrast, diets heavy in refined carbohydrates, saturated fats, and processed foods have been related to an elevated risk of mood disorders and psychological discomfort.

According to a new study, the gut microbiota plays an important role in the bidirectional communication between the stomach and the brain, known as the gut-brain axis. Disruptions in gut microbiota composition, which are often caused by poor food choices and lifestyle variables, have been related to changes in mood, cognition, and behavior, emphasizing the significance of a good diet in promoting mental health and emotional wellbeing.

Importance of Individualized Nutrition

Individual reactions to nutrition vary greatly depending on heredity, metabolism, lifestyle, and underlying health issues.

Certain eating habits may be advantageous to one individual but not necessarily ideal for another. Personalized nutrition strategies that include individual requirements, preferences, and objectives are critical for improving health outcomes and fostering long-term wellbeing.

A diversified diet rich in whole foods from all food categories contains a wide range of vital nutrients and phytonutrients, which promotes general health and reduces the risk of nutritional shortages. Incorporating a colorful array of fruits, vegetables, whole grains, lean meats, and healthy fats into daily meals guarantees a balanced intake of important nutrients while also encouraging dietary diversity and pleasure.

Mindful eating techniques that encourage awareness, presence, and intentionality in food intake may help people have a healthy connection with food, increase pleasure and enjoyment, and improve overall wellbeing. Mindful eating entails hunger and fullness signals, relishing food tastes and textures, and cultivating a nonjudgmental attitude toward eating behaviors and food choices.

Finally, nutrition has a substantial and diverse influence on total health, affecting physiological, psychological, and emotional wellbeing. A healthy diet high in essential nutrients, balanced macronutrients, and hydration promotes optimal metabolic function, disease prevention, and mental health. In contrast, personalized nutrition approaches and mindful eating practices enable people to make informed decisions based on their specific needs and goals. Prioritizing nutritional quality, variety, and awareness allows us to nurture our bodies, minds, and spirits, cultivating a foundation of health and vitality that enhances all parts of our lives.

The Role of Organic Foods in Disease Prevention

Diet is a significant predictor of health outcomes in the context of illness prevention. As we traverse the intricacies of contemporary food production and consumption, the decision between organic and conventional foods becomes more important, with organic foods gaining popularity due to their possible health advantages. In this chapter, we will look at how organic foods may help prevent illness, how they affect critical health outcomes, and what scientific data supports their usefulness.

Understanding organic foods

Organic foods are grown using agricultural techniques that promote soil health, biodiversity, and ecological balance while limiting the use of synthetic chemicals, pesticides, and genetically modified organisms (GMOs). Organic farmers use a range of sustainable strategies, including crop rotation, cover cropping, and natural pest management, to improve soil fertility and plant health without depending on chemicals.

Organic foods must meet severe certification and labeling criteria set by regulatory authorities such as the United States Department of Agriculture (USDA) and the European Union. These standards specify the techniques and chemicals that may be used in the manufacturing, processing, and labeling of organic foods, providing transparency and integrity across the supply chain.

Organic foods are often lauded for their improved nutritional profile, with research indicating that they may contain greater quantities of key elements such as vitamins, minerals, antioxidants, and phytonutrients than conventionally cultivated competitors. Organic fruits, vegetables, cereals, and dairy products are also free of synthetic pesticides and chemicals, lowering exposure to potentially dangerous substances while increasing general health and wellbeing.

The Effect of Organic Foods on Disease Prevention

Numerous studies have looked at the link between organic food intake and cardiovascular health outcomes, with findings indicating that organic diets may be connected with a lower risk of heart disease, stroke, and hypertension. Organic foods are often lower in saturated fats and richer in heart-healthy elements, including omega-3 fatty acids, antioxidants, and phytonutrients, which may aid in decreasing cholesterol, reducing inflammation, and enhancing vascular function.

Organic meat and dairy products from pasture-raised animals have more omega-3 fatty acids, including eicosapentaenoic acid (EPA) and docosahexaenoic acid (DHA), which have been demonstrated to improve cardiovascular health. Omega-3 fatty acids decrease triglyceride levels, lower blood pressure, and enhance endothelial function, all of which lessen the risk of heart disease and stroke.

Organic fruits and vegetables include high levels of antioxidants, including vitamin C, vitamin E, and polyphenols, which aid in neutralizing free radicals and minimize oxidative stress in the body. Antioxidants have been associated with a reduced risk of cardiovascular disease because they protect against lipid oxidation, inflammation, and endothelial dysfunction.

The possible significance of organic foods in cancer prevention has been investigated scientifically, with studies indicating that organic diets may be connected with a lower risk of some forms of cancer. Organic foods do not include synthetic pesticides, herbicides, or genetically modified organisms (GMOs), all of which have been linked to cancer and tumor formation. Organic foods are less likely to contain pesticide residues than conventionally cultivated foods, which reduces exposure to potentially carcinogenic substances.

According to studies, those who are exposed to more pesticides are more likely to get specific malignancies, such as leukemia, lymphoma, breast cancer, and prostate cancer. Organic fruits and vegetables include more bioactive components, such as flavonoids, phenolic acids, and glucosinolates, which have been found to have anticarcinogenic effects. These substances aid in inhibiting tumor growth, suppressing cancer cell proliferation, and inducing apoptosis (programmed cell death), lowering the risk of cancer formation and progression.

Emerging research shows that organic foods may help to promote neurological health and cognitive function, with studies revealing a possible relationship between organic food intake and a lower risk of neurodegenerative disorders, including Alzheimer's and Parkinson's. Organic foods do not contain synthetic pesticides or chemicals, which have been linked to neurotoxicity and cognitive impairment. Pesticide exposure has been linked to neurological illnesses such as Parkinson's disease, Alzheimer's disease, and cognitive loss, especially in sensitive groups such as children and the elderly.

Organic fruits and vegetables have high levels of antioxidants, including vitamin C, vitamin E, and polyphenols, which assist in protecting the brain from oxidative stress and inflammation. Antioxidants have been demonstrated to promote brain health, increase cognitive performance, and lower the risk of age-related neurodegenerative disorders.

Organic foods also help to improve immune function and reduce the risk of infectious illnesses by supplying critical nutrients and promoting general health and wellness. Organic foods are frequently richer in critical elements, including vitamins, minerals, and antioxidants, which are necessary for a healthy immune system. Nutrient shortages may weaken immunological responses and increase susceptibility to infections, while an immune-boosting diet strengthens immune defenses and increases resistance to pathogens.

Organic foods promote a healthy gut microbiome, which is a varied collection of bacteria found in the gastrointestinal system and plays an important role in immunological function. Fiber-rich, fermented, and prebiotic-rich foods included in organic diets encourage the development of good gut bacteria and contribute to a healthy microbial environment, lowering the risk of infectious illnesses and increasing immunological resilience.

The Organic Diet and Weight Management

In the never-ending pursuit of weight loss and general wellbeing, the organic diet has emerged as an appealing strategy that prioritizes food quality and sources above calorie tracking. This chapter will investigate the complex link between the organic diet and weight control, investigating the ways by which organic foods may impact body weight, metabolic health, and general wellbeing.

Understanding the organic diet

The organic diet is founded on concepts of sustainability, environmental care, and overall wellness. It stresses eating whole, minimally processed foods devoid of synthetic pesticides, herbicides, fertilizers, and genetically modified organisms (GMOs). Organic farming approaches promote soil health, biodiversity, and ecological balance, boosting agricultural system sustainability and minimizing industrial agriculture's negative environmental consequences.

Organic foods are often lauded for their improved nutritional profile, with research indicating that they may contain greater quantities of key elements such as vitamins, minerals, antioxidants, and phytonutrients than conventionally cultivated competitors. Organic fruits, vegetables, cereals, and dairy products are also free of synthetic pesticides and chemicals, lowering exposure to potentially dangerous substances while increasing general health and wellbeing.

The Role of Organic Diets in Weight Management

One of the primary ways that the organic diet may impact weight control is via its concentration of nutrient-dense foods that promote satiety and pleasure. Organic fruits, vegetables, whole grains, and lean meats are high in important nutrients and fiber, which help control hunger, balance blood sugar levels, and avoid overeating. Organic foods are frequently richer in fiber than conventionally cultivated foods, owing to changes in agricultural techniques and soil management.

Fiber promotes feelings of fullness and satiety, reduces appetite and cravings, and aids in weight control by limiting overeating and improving calorie balance. The higher nutritional profile of organic foods may also improve nutrient absorption and utilization, enabling the body to get the most advantage from the foods ingested. Adequate consumption of vital nutrients such as vitamins, minerals, and antioxidants is critical for sustaining metabolic function, energy generation, and general wellbeing, all of which are important components of effective weight control.

Another possible advantage of the organic diet for weight loss is lower exposure to synthetic chemicals, pesticides, and additives present in conventionally cultivated foods. Organic agricultural techniques ban the use of synthetic pesticides and chemicals, reducing the possibility of chemical residues in food and the environment. Synthetic pesticides and chemicals used in traditional agriculture have been linked to hormonal imbalances and metabolic disturbances, which may lead to weight gain and obesity. Some pesticides have been proven to disrupt thyroid function, insulin sensitivity, and adipocyte (fat cell) metabolism, possibly resulting in metabolic dysregulation and weight-related health concerns. Exposure to synthetic hormones, antibiotics, and growth promoters, which are widely used in traditional animal husbandry, has also been linked to hormonal imbalance and weight gain. Hormones like estrogen, progesterone, and testosterone regulate metabolism, appetite, and fat storage, and hormonal imbalances may lead to weight-related problems, including insulin resistance, leptin resistance, and metabolic syndrome.

The organic diet benefits not only human health but also environmental sustainability, which might have an indirect impact on weight control results. Organic farming techniques improve soil health, biodiversity, and ecological balance, all of which are critical for sustaining the planet's health and guaranteeing a reliable food supply for future generations. Industrial agriculture, which includes heavy chemical inputs, monoculture farming, and deforestation, contributes significantly to climate change and environmental damage.

Organic agriculture, on the other hand, helps to reduce climate change by sequestering carbon in the soil, lowering greenhouse gas emissions, and protecting natural ecosystems. Organic agriculture promotes sustainable food systems that encourage local food production, seasonal eating, and decreased food waste, which may have a good impact on weight control and general health. Organic diets promote healthy eating habits and lifestyle choices that aid in weight control and long-term wellbeing by increasing access to fresh, nutritious foods while decreasing dependence on processed and packaged goods.

Challenges and considerations

While the organic diet has many potential advantages for weight control and general health, it has its drawbacks and concerns. Accessibility, cost, and availability of organic foods may be challenges for certain people, especially those who live in food deserts or low-income neighborhoods.

Organic foods may be more costly and less readily available than conventionally cultivated competitors, making it difficult for some people to integrate organic foods into their diet on a regular basis. The need for more organic products in some geographic locations or retail settings may create hurdles to entry for customers looking to embrace an organic lifestyle.

The apparent high cost of organic foods may dissuade some people from adopting them into their diet, especially those on a tight budget or fixed income. While organic foods may be more expensive than conventionally produced alternatives, the long-term health advantages and possible cost savings associated with lower healthcare bills and better general wellbeing may exceed the initial investment in organic foods.

Organic food availability varies according to geographic area, seasonality, and retail distribution methods. While organic alternatives are becoming more common in conventional grocery stores, specialized markets, and farmers' markets, customers in specific regions or rural areas may need more access to organic goods, making it difficult to stick to an organic diet regularly.

Adopting an organic diet offers a diverse approach to improving overall health and wellbeing, taking into account physiological, psychological, and environmental factors. Individuals who prioritize nutrient-dense meals farmed without synthetic pesticides or genetically modified organisms may be able to minimize their risk of a variety of chronic illnesses while also fostering optimum metabolic and mental health. Furthermore, organic farming techniques help to ensure environmental sustainability by protecting soil health, biodiversity, and animal welfare, which aligns with social responsibility values. However, some people may find it difficult to follow an organic diet due to factors such as accessibility and cost.

Nonetheless, continued efforts to increase access to organic foods and educate the public about their advantages are critical steps toward breaking down these barriers and fostering better eating habits and sustainable food systems for everyone. In essence, the organic diet is a lifestyle choice that prioritizes the wellbeing of our bodies, brains, and the environment. As we continue to investigate the relationship between nutrition, health, and environmental sustainability, the adoption of organic foods appears as a possible route toward a better, healthier future for people and communities globally.

In Chapter 3, we'll look at the functions of macronutrients (carbs, proteins, and fats) and micronutrients (vitamins and minerals) in sustaining health. Macronutrients provide energy and raw materials, while micronutrients aid physiological processes. Balanced nutrition derived from entire meals is essential, with plant-based alternatives giving antioxidants and animal-based ones supplying protein. Understanding and balancing these nutrients improves metabolic health and illness prevention. In addition, we'll discuss the advantages of absorbing important nutrients from organic sources, stressing their superior nutritional value. Finally, meal planning techniques will be reviewed to provide a varied and fulfilling diet that meets individual dietary requirements and promotes overall wellbeing.

Chapter 3

Macro and Micronutrient Overview

In the complicated dance of nutrition, macronutrients, and micronutrients take center stage as critical components of a balanced diet that feeds our bodies and promotes maximum health and wellbeing. In this chapter, we will explore the interesting world of macro and micronutrients, investigating their functions, sources, and significance in sustaining a balanced diet and lifestyle.

Understanding macro and micronutrients

Macronutrients are the fundamental components of our food, supplying the energy and raw materials required for growth, development, and metabolic function. There are three types of macronutrients: carbs, proteins, and lipids, each with a distinct function in supporting physiological processes and providing the body's energy requirements.

Carbohydrates are the body's major source of energy, fueling cellular metabolism, physical activity, and mental function. Carbs are present in a wide range of foods, including fruits, vegetables, grains, legumes, and dairy products. Complex carbs, such as whole grains and starchy vegetables, provide continuous energy and fiber for digestive health.

Proteins are required for tissue repair, muscular development, immunological function, and hormone production, as well as the formation of enzymes, antibodies, and structural components of cells and tissues. Meat, poultry, fish, eggs, dairy products, legumes, nuts, and seeds are examples of protein-rich diets. Complete proteins include all of the essential amino acids required for human health.

Fats are a concentrated source of energy and critical fatty acids, with important roles in cell membrane formation, hormone synthesis, nutrition absorption, and insulation. Healthy fats include monounsaturated fats like olive oil, avocados, and almonds, polyunsaturated fats like fatty fish, flaxseeds, and walnuts, and omega-3 fatty acids like fish oil, algal oil, and flaxseed oil.

Micronutrients are vitamins and minerals that are necessary in trace levels for a variety of physiological processes such as enzyme functioning, metabolism, immunological function, and bone health. Micronutrients are present in a variety of foods, including fruits, vegetables, whole grains, lean proteins, and dairy products, and they play an important role in general health and wellness.

Vitamins are chemical substances that serve as coenzymes or cofactors in metabolic processes, promoting energy generation, antioxidant protection, and immunological function. There are 13 important vitamins, including vitamin A, vitamin C, vitamin D, vitamin E, and the B-complex vitamins (B1, B2, B3, B5, B6, B7, B9, and B12), each having a distinct purpose and function in the body.

Minerals are:

Inorganic elements that operate as structural components of bones and teeth.

- Electrolytes for fluid balance and nerve function.
- Cofactors for enzyme activity and cell metabolism.

Calcium, magnesium, phosphorus, potassium, sodium, chloride, iron, zinc, selenium, copper, manganese, iodine, and chromium are all essential minerals that help maintain physiological homeostasis and promote general health.

The importance of macro and micronutrients in the diet

Macronutrients, such as carbs, proteins, and lipids, provide the energy required for cellular metabolism, physical activity, and cognitive function. Carbohydrates are the body's principal source of energy, although proteins and fats act as alternate fuel sources and play essential roles in energy metabolism and storage.

Proteins, vitamins, and minerals are required for normal growth, development, and tissue repair, as well as muscle growth, bone production, and immunological function. Adequate protein, calcium, vitamin D, and other micronutrient consumption is especially critical during times of fast growth and development, such as childhood, adolescence, pregnancy, and breastfeeding.

Micronutrients such as vitamins A, C, D, E, and zinc are essential for immunological function and disease prevention. These vitamins and minerals assist in boosting the immune system, control inflammation, and improve the body's capacity to combat diseases and external invaders.

Macro and micronutrients play important roles in regulating metabolism, blood sugar levels, and hormone balance. These are necessary for metabolic health and the prevention of chronic illnesses, including obesity, type 2 diabetes, and metabolic syndrome. Nutrient-dense diets, including fruits, vegetables, whole grains, and lean meats, boost metabolic function and general health.

Dietary sources of macro- and micronutrients

Whole foods, including fruits, vegetables, whole grains, lean meats, and dairy products, are high in macro and micronutrients, offering a wide range of vital nutrients in their natural form. These nutrient-dense foods should serve as the cornerstone of a balanced diet, providing the building blocks for overall health and wellbeing.

Plant-based foods, including fruits, vegetables, legumes, nuts, and seeds, are high in vitamins, minerals, antioxidants, and phytonutrients. These help with immune function, cardiovascular health, and general wellbeing. Plant-based diets are linked to a variety of health advantages, including lower risk of chronic illnesses, better weight control, and increased lifespan.

Animal-based foods, such as meat, chicken, fish, eggs, and dairy products, include high-quality protein, vitamins, and minerals required for muscular development, bone health, and metabolism. While animal-based meals may supply key nutrients, it is critical to pick lean protein sources and limit your consumption of saturated fats and processed meats to maintain heart health and general wellbeing.

Balance Macronutrients and Micronutrients in the Diet

The Dietary Guidelines for Americans encourage a well-balanced diet rich in nutrients from all food categories, such as fruits, vegetables, whole grains, lean meats, and dairy products. The recommendations highlight the necessity of ingesting a diverse range of macronutrients and micronutrients to satisfy nutritional requirements and promote overall health and wellbeing.

Portion management is essential for balancing macronutrient and micronutrient consumption while maintaining a healthy weight and lifestyle. By regulating portion sizes and calorie consumption, individuals may achieve their nutritional requirements while avoiding overeating and supporting weight management.

Eating a comprehensive and varied diet that includes foods from all food categories offers a balanced macronutrient and micronutrient intake while also supporting general health and wellbeing. Individuals may enhance their nutritional status by including a colorful variety of fruits and vegetables, whole grains, lean meats, and healthy fats in meals and snacks.

It's important to understand that individual nutritional requirements might vary depending on age, gender, exercise level, and health state. Customizing the diet to match personal needs and tastes ensures that dietary requirements are satisfied while also supporting optimum health and wellbeing throughout the life cycle.

Including Essential Nutrients from Organic Sources

In the quest for maximum health and wellbeing, the source of our nutrition is critical. Organic foods, grown using sustainable agricultural techniques and devoid of synthetic chemicals and pesticides, have gained popularity due to their ability to deliver essential nutrients while reducing exposure to dangerous substances. In this chapter, we'll look at the abundance of critical nutrients present in organic foods and discuss how to include them in a healthy diet.

Understanding the Essential Nutrients

Essential nutrients include a wide range of macro and micronutrients required to maintain life and promote health. Macronutrients, such as carbohydrates, proteins, and fats, provide energy and structural components, while micronutrients, such as vitamins and minerals, control biochemical processes and support physiological activities.

Essential nutrients are important in many aspects of human physiology, including energy metabolism, tissue regeneration, immunological function, and cognitive functioning. Adequate nutrition is vital for maintaining good health and wellbeing, promoting growth and development, and lowering the risk of chronic illnesses.

Nutrient Density in Organic Foods

Organic foods are known for their enhanced nutritional profile, with research indicating that they may contain more critical elements than conventionally farmed alternatives. Organic fruits, vegetables, cereals, and dairy products include a high concentration of vitamins, minerals, antioxidants, and phytonutrients, all of which promote overall health and wellness.

Organic fruits and vegetables are especially high in antioxidants, which help neutralize free radicals and minimize oxidative stress in the body. Antioxidants, including vitamin C, vitamin E, and polyphenols, help protect cells from harm, boost immunological function, and lower the risk of chronic illnesses.

Including Essential Nutrients from Organic Sources

Incorporating a variety of organic fruits and vegetables into meals and snacks provides a wide range of critical nutrients and phytonutrients. Aim for a spectrum of hues, including brilliant greens, reds, oranges, yellows, and blues, to increase nutrient intake and boost general wellness. Buying organic fruits and vegetables in season assures freshness, taste, and nutritional value. Seasonal eating also promotes environmental sustainability by minimizing the carbon footprint of food transportation and increasing biodiversity in local food systems.

Choose organic whole grains like brown rice, quinoa, oats, barley, and whole wheat, which preserve their natural bran, germ, and endosperm while also providing fiber, vitamins, minerals, and phytonutrients in plenty. Whole grains give long-lasting energy, boost digestive health, and improve cardiovascular health. Explore ancient grains, including amaranth, farro, millet, and teff, which have distinct aromas, textures, and nutritional profiles. Ancient grains are high in protein, fiber, and important elements, and they are often grown utilizing traditional and sustainable agricultural methods.

Choose organic meat and poultry from pasture-raised animals that have not received antibiotics, hormones, or synthetic growth boosters. Organic beef and poultry are low in fat and high in critical minerals like iron, zinc, and B vitamins, all of which promote muscular building, immunological function, and general health. Choose organic and sustainably obtained seafood, such as wild-caught fish and shellfish, which are high in omega-3 fatty acids, protein, and other minerals. Organic seafood promotes marine conservation and lowers the environmental effects of aquaculture methods.

Choose organic dairy products like milk, yogurt, and cheese made from grass-fed cows that are free of synthetic hormones and antibiotics. Organic dairy products are high in calcium, protein, and vital vitamins like vitamin D and B12, which help with bone health, muscular function, and general wellbeing. Investigate organic plant-based alternatives to dairy products, including almond milk, coconut yogurt, and cashew cheese, which provide dairy-free choices for anyone with lactose sensitivity or dietary restrictions. Plant-based alternatives are high in vitamins, minerals, and antioxidants and may be used in a wide range of recipes and gourmet creations.

Maximizing Nutritional Benefits

To keep organic foods nutritionally intact and improve nutrient absorption, use moderate cooking techniques such as steaming, roasting, and sautéing. Avoid high temperatures and extensive cooking periods, which might damage heat-sensitive vitamins and antioxidants. Combining organic meals with complementary substances improves nutrient absorption and bioavailability. For example, combining vitamin C-rich fruits and vegetables with iron-rich plant meals or lean meats may improve iron absorption while also supporting immunological function and energy metabolism.

Savor each mouthful, chew gently, and be aware of hunger and fullness signs. Mindful eating encourages awareness, pleasure, and contentment with food, which leads to better digestion, less overeating, and better nutritional absorption. Make conscientious eating choices that emphasize nutrient-dense organic foods and promote general health and wellbeing. Consider the environmental, ethical, and social aspects of food production and consumption, and choose organic choices that are consistent with your particular beliefs and aspirations.

Meal Planning and Balanced Nutrition

Meal planning is an essential step in achieving balanced nutrition and maintaining good health and wellbeing. Individuals may achieve their overall health objectives by carefully choosing a range of nutrient-dense foods and combining them into well-balanced meals and snacks. In this chapter, we will look at meal planning concepts and how to prepare balanced meals with vital nutrients from a range of food sources.

Understand Meal Planning

Meal planning is carefully selecting foods and recipes to produce balanced meals and snacks that fit individual nutritional requirements and tastes. It is an important tool for encouraging good eating habits, reducing dietary shortages, and improving general health and wellbeing. Meal planning ensures that people eat a healthy balance of macronutrients and micronutrients. Individuals may achieve their nutritional demands by including a range of nutrient-dense foods in their meals and snacks while also supporting metabolic function, energy generation, and immunological function.

Meal planning may help people save time and money by decreasing food waste, limiting grocery shop excursions, and optimizing food budgets. Individuals may save time and money on food by planning meals and preparing materials ahead of time. Meal planning promotes nutritional diversity by combining a wide range of foods from all food categories into meals and snacks. Individuals may broaden their culinary expertise, explore new tastes and textures, and enjoy a more diverse and fulfilling diet by rotating food options and experimenting with different recipes.

Principles of Balanced Nutrition

Incorporate complex carbs such as whole grains, fruits, vegetables, and legumes into your meals and snacks to give long-lasting energy and fiber for digestive health. Include a variety of colorful fruits and vegetables in your meals to increase nutritional intake and boost overall health. Include lean protein sources in your meals, such as fowl, fish, tofu, beans, and lentils, to promote muscle development, tissue repair, and immunological function. To achieve a balanced intake of essential amino acids, spread protein consumption equally throughout the day and mix up protein sources. Incorporate healthy fats like olive oil, avocados, nuts, and seeds into your meals and snacks to improve cardiovascular health, cognitive function, and hormone balance. Limit your consumption of saturated and trans fats found in fried meals, processed snacks, and fatty meats since they may lead to heart disease and metabolic dysfunction.

Choose nutrient-dense meals like fruits, vegetables, whole grains, lean meats, and dairy products to acquire the important vitamins and minerals you need for good health. Include a diversity of colors, textures, and tastes in your meals to increase nutrient intake and enhance overall nutritional sufficiency. Choose foods high in antioxidants and phytonutrients, such as berries, leafy greens, cruciferous vegetables, and herbs and spices, to boost immune function, decrease inflammation, and protect against chronic illnesses. Incorporate a variety of colored fruits and vegetables into your meals to increase antioxidant consumption and enhance cellular health.

Include fiber-rich foods in your meals and snacks to improve digestive health, control blood sugar levels, and increase satiety. Consume a variety of soluble and insoluble fiber sources to improve overall gastrointestinal function and regularity. Drink lots of water throughout the day, and include hydrating items like fruits, vegetables, soups, and herbal teas in your meals and snacks. Aim to drink at least eight glasses of water every day and vary fluid consumption depending on personal hydration requirements, activity level, and ambient circumstances.

Practical Strategies for Meal Planning

Determine particular health goals and priorities, such as weight management, blood sugar control, or cardiovascular health, and customize meal planning efforts to meet these goals. Consider speaking with a certified dietician or healthcare practitioner for tailored advice and assistance. When planning meals and snacks, consider individual nutritional preferences, cultural customs, and lifestyle concerns. Include a range of flavors, textures, and cuisines in meal planning to cater to different tastes and preferences.

Set aside time each week to establish a food plan that includes breakfast, lunch, supper, and snacks for each day. To keep meals interesting and pleasurable, try combining classic favorites with new ones. Spending time batch cooking and prepping items ahead of time may simplify meal preparation and save time during busier weekdays. Cook grains, slice veggies, and divide out meats to make ready-to-eat ingredients that may be quickly combined into meals throughout the week.

Create a shopping list based on the items required for the week's meals and snacks, and stick to it when grocery shopping to avoid impulsive purchases and ensure you have everything you need to create healthy meals at home. Fill your shopping basket with nutrient-dense foods like fruits, vegetables, whole grains, lean meats, and dairy products to ensure you receive the vitamins, minerals, and antioxidants you need for good health.

Finally, knowing the role of macronutrients and micronutrients in our diet is critical for improving overall health and wellness. Individuals who understand the roles and sources of these vital nutrients may make educated choices to guarantee appropriate nutrition and support their long-term health objectives.

Macro and micronutrients are engaged in a variety of physiological processes, ranging from energy generation to immune function, emphasizing the need for a nutrient-dense diet for overall health and vitality.

Incorporating nutrients from organic sources improves the health advantages of a balanced diet. Individuals who prioritize organic foods such as fruits, vegetables, whole grains, lean proteins, and dairy products might not only satisfy their nutritional requirements but may also benefit from extra physiological, environmental, and social benefits. Organic foods include more antioxidants and help to create sustainable food systems that are consistent with health, environmental stewardship, and social responsibility values.

Meal planning emerges as a viable technique for achieving balanced nutrition and promoting overall health. By adopting a range of nutrient-dense foods, individuals may reach their nutritional needs while still enjoying good and gratifying meals and snacks. Meal planning enables people to take charge of their nutrition, make educated food choices, and nurture their bodies and souls properly. Thus, adopting balanced nutrition and meal planning encourages a holistic approach to health, which improves quality of life and general wellbeing.

Embrace the organic revolution! Transitioning to an organic diet is a worthwhile process, which includes selecting pesticide-free vegetables and discovering local farmers' markets. With each step, you are not only fueling your body with nutritious foods but also promoting sustainable agriculture and environmental health. Overcome obstacles by purchasing wisely, eating seasonally, and even planting your organic garden. Prioritizing health, sustainability, and resilience does more than change your diet; it also changes the globe, one organic decision at a time. So, let us go on this organic journey together, making conscientious decisions that benefit both ourselves and the environment. Join the movement, and let's grow organically.

Chapter 4

A Transition to an Organic Lifestyle

Transitioning to an organic lifestyle marks a significant transformation in our attitude toward food, health, and environmental sustainability. It entails not just modifying what we eat but also rethinking our relationship with food, promoting sustainable agriculture methods, and putting our health and wellbeing first. In this chapter, we will look at the strategies and tactics for transitioning to an organic lifestyle, from comprehending the advantages of organic foods to practical advice for integrating organic choices into your everyday life.

Understanding the benefits of organic food

Organic foods are grown using sustainable agricultural techniques that do not allow the use of synthetic pesticides, herbicides, or fertilizers. Individuals who choose organic products may lower their exposure to potentially dangerous chemicals as well as the possibility of pesticide residues in food and water. According to studies, organic foods may include more critical elements such as vitamins, minerals, antioxidants, and phytonutrients than conventionally cultivated competitors. Organic fruits, vegetables, cereals, and dairy products contain a high concentration of important nutrients that promote overall health and wellness. Eating organic foods has been linked to a decreased risk of chronic illnesses, including obesity, type 2 diabetes, cardiovascular disease, and several forms of cancer. Organic foods are free of synthetic chemicals and pesticides, which may assist in decreasing inflammation, improving immunological function, protecting against oxidative stress, and encouraging long-term health and wellbeing.

Organic farming approaches promote soil health, biodiversity, and ecological balance, boosting agricultural system sustainability and minimizing industrial agriculture's negative environmental consequences. Individuals who choose organic foods may help to promote sustainable food systems that conserve natural ecosystems and ensure the planet's health for future generations. Crop rotation, composting, and integrated pest management are examples of organic farming strategies that help trap carbon in the soil, decrease greenhouse gas emissions, and mitigate climate change. Individuals who support organic agriculture may help to battle global climate change and promote environmental sustainability.

Steps to Transition to an Organic Lifestyle

Familiarize yourself with the rules and laws that govern organic certification, such as organic agricultural techniques, labeling, and certification procedures. To understand more about the advantages and principles of organic agriculture, consult credible websites, nonprofit organizations, and government authorities. Familiarize yourself with the Environmental Working Group's (EWG) "Dirty Dozen" and "Clean Fifteen" lists, which rate the fruits and vegetables with the most and least pesticide residues. Use this information to prioritize organic choices for the most pesticide-contaminated crops.

Begin by emphasizing organic choices for pesticide-contaminated foods such as fruits, vegetables, dairy products, and meat. Begin by introducing organic versions of your favorite fruits and veggies into meals and snacks, gradually increasing your organic options over time. Transition to an organic diet by focusing on organic basics, including grains, beans, nuts, seeds, oils, and spices, which serve as the basis for many meals and dishes. Look for organic alternatives to cupboard essentials like rice, pasta, beans, and cooking oils to maintain a steady supply of organic items in your kitchen.

When shopping for organic foods, carefully examine the labels to confirm that the items are certified organic by a reputable certifying agency. Look for the USDA Organic label or other credible organic certification logo on the packaging to ensure that the food meets organic criteria and contains at least 95% organic components. Visit local farmers' markets, co-ops, and organic grocery shops to find a diverse range of organic vegetables, dairy products, meats, and pantry necessities. Support local farmers and producers by buying organic products from small-scale, sustainable businesses that value organic agricultural techniques and environmental management.

Embrace the changing seasons by including seasonal fruits and vegetables in your meals and snacks. Choose organic seasonal vegetables whenever feasible, and find new ways to enjoy the tastes and textures of fresh, locally produced foods all year. Take advantage of seasonal bounty by preserving and storing fresh fruits and vegetables for future use. Experiment with home canning, freezing, drying, and fermentation methods to prolong the shelf life of seasonal vegetables and enjoy summer tastes all year long.

Consider developing a home garden to produce your organic fruits, veggies, herbs, and spices. Whether you have a little balcony, backyard, or communal plot, gardening allows you to connect with nature, raise your food, and experience the pleasure of reaping fresh products. Composting, mulching, companion planting, and natural pest control are all organic gardening strategies that help you maintain a healthy and productive garden without using synthetic chemicals or pesticides. Create a diversified and resilient ecosystem that sustains beneficial insects, pollinators, and soil microbes while also promoting plant and human health.

Overcoming Challenges

Recognize that organic goods may cost more than conventionally cultivated equivalents owing to increased manufacturing costs and certification requirements. Prioritize organic choices for pesticide-contaminated foods and search for cost-saving techniques like purchasing in bulk, shopping discounts, and joining a CSA (Community Supported Agriculture) program to save costs.

Recognize that access to organic foods might vary based on geography, availability, and resources. To expand your organic food choices and support local farmers, look into alternate sources such as internet shops, farm-to-table delivery services, and community food cooperatives.

Lisa, a single mom with a demanding schedule, struggled to find time for food planning and preparation. She was first intimidated by the prospect of adopting an organic lifestyle, but she was determined to make a good difference for herself and her children. Lisa sought the assistance of a nutritionist, who offered practical advice on meal planning, bulk cooking, and introducing organic foods into her family's diet. Lisa progressively adopted an organic lifestyle with support and coaching, resulting in improvements in her energy levels, mood, and general wellbeing.

Adopting a holistic approach

Practice mindful eating by enjoying each mouthful, paying attention to hunger and fullness signals, and being grateful for the nutrition supplied by organic foods. Slow down, focus your senses, and enjoy the tastes, textures, and fragrances of fresh, healthful meals while nourishing your body and spirit. Spending time outside, visiting local parks, gardens, and nature reserves, and enjoying the earth's beauty and richness can help you reconnect with nature. Develop a stronger connection to the land, the seasons, and the natural cycles of life, and recognize the interdependence of all living species.

David, a holistic health coach, underlined the significance of mindfulness and connection in the shift to an organic lifestyle. David encouraged his customers to become more conscious of their food choices and their influence on health and the environment by including activities like mindful eating, gratitude journaling, and nature excursions. David's customers felt more satisfied, fulfilled, and vital in their transition to an organic lifestyle because he fostered a feeling of connection with nature and the food they ate.

Overcoming Challenges and Obstacles.

Transitioning to an organic lifestyle is a pleasant path toward greater health, environmental sustainability, and ethical eating habits. However, like with any substantial shift, there will be hurdles and impediments. In this chapter, we'll look at major roadblocks that people may experience while adopting an organic lifestyle and present practical techniques and real-life examples for overcoming them.

Understanding the Common Challenges

One of the most frequent obstacles people face when shifting to an organic diet is the notion that organic products are more expensive than traditionally grown ones. Smaller-scale manufacturing, certification procedures, and restricted availability all contribute to the higher prices of organic goods.

Access to organic foods may vary based on geographic location, socioeconomic level, and the availability of organic products at local grocery shops and marketplaces. Individuals living in rural or low-income regions may need help accessing organic items or have restricted transportation alternatives to reach organic food sources.

People may need to become more familiar with the concepts of organic agriculture, the advantages of organic foods, and how to recognize organic goods. If they lack this knowledge and information, they may feel overwhelmed or unsure about making educated decisions regarding organic eating.

Individuals who want to emphasize organic food may need help due to their busy lives, demanding schedules, and time limits. Meal planning, shopping for organic goods, and making meals from scratch may entail extra time and effort that many may need help to fit into their regular schedules.

Practical Strategies for Overcoming Challenges

Identify high-impact foods with the most pesticide contamination, such as fruits and vegetables, from the Environmental Working Group's "Dirty Dozen" list, and favor organic alternatives. Individuals should spend their food budget and reduce pesticide exposure by concentrating on crucial purchases. Look for ways to save money, such as purchasing in bulk, taking advantage of deals and promotions, joining a community-supported agriculture (CSA) program, or joining a food cooperative. These solutions may help people save money on organic foods, making them cheaper and more accessible.

If you have limited access to organic goods in your region, look into alternate sources, including farmers' markets, co-ops, internet sellers, and community-supported agriculture (CSA) programs. These choices may give a more diverse variety of organic items as well as possibilities to contact directly with local farmers and producers. If your town needs access to organic goods, try lobbying for change by contacting local legislators, community groups, and grocery stores. Raise awareness about the need for organic alternatives and push for programs like farmers' markets, urban gardens, and organic food cooperatives to promote access to organic foods for all citizens.

Take the time to learn about the principles of organic agriculture, the advantages of organic foods, and how to recognize organic goods. Use materials such as books, websites, videos, and online courses to get a better knowledge of organic agricultural techniques and the necessity of sustainable food systems. Share your organic food knowledge and observations with friends, family, and community members to increase awareness and support educated eating choices. Organize educational events, culinary classes, or documentary screenings to start discussions about the advantages of organic eating and motivate people to choose healthier, more sustainable food choices.

Set aside time each week to plan meals, make shopping lists, and prep items in advance to simplify meal preparation and reduce time spent in the kitchen. Use meal planning apps, internet tools, and cookbooks to get ideas and streamline the meal planning process. On weekends or days off, spend time batch cooking and meal preparing to prepare ingredients, cook dishes in bulk, then divide out portions for convenient reheating throughout the week.

Invest in storage containers, reusable bags, and meal prep accessories to help you organize your supplies and speed up the meal preparation process.

David and Lisa, a busy couple combining work and family commitments, struggled to make time for food preparation and cooking throughout the week. They established a Sunday meal prep schedule in which they spent a few hours preparing huge amounts of grains, meats, and veggies to serve as the basis for meals during the week. By preparing ingredients ahead of time and keeping them in portioned containers, David and Lisa were able to save time and enjoy delicious, home-cooked meals without having to cook from scratch every day.

Cultivating resilience and persistence

Transitioning to an organic lifestyle needs strength, perseverance, and dedication. Regardless of the problems and hurdles that may occur, it is important to keep focused on your objectives, appreciate minor triumphs, and be open to learning and growing along the way. By adopting a resilient and persistent mentality, you may overcome obstacles, handle setbacks, and continue on your journey to health, sustainability, and wellbeing.

Michelle, a single mom juggling her job and family duties, had various hurdles when transitioning to an organic lifestyle. Despite the restricted availability of organic goods and time restrictions, Michelle stayed determined to prioritize organic alternatives for her family. She sought encouragement from online forums and engaged in culinary lessons. She tried out different recipes and cooking methods to help her overcome challenges and remain on track with her organic path. Michelle successfully switched her family to an organic diet, and their health and wellbeing improved significantly as a result of her effort and drive.

Tips for Maintaining Motivation

Transitioning to an organic lifestyle entails more than simply altering your diet; it requires a complete adjustment in mentality and practices toward health, sustainability, and ethical consumerism. While the initial exhilaration of starting this trip might generate impetus, maintaining motivation over time can be difficult. In this chapter, we'll look at practical advice and tactics for staying motivated on your organic lifestyle journey.

Sustaining motivation is critical for long-term success in adopting and living an organic lifestyle. It enables people to remain dedicated to their objectives, overcome obstacles, and accept the adjustments required to attain health, sustainability, and wellbeing. Motivation is essential in incorporating organic food into everyday life as a sustainable and joyful lifestyle option. Individuals who remain motivated may develop long-term routines and behaviors that benefit their health, the environment, and ethical eating choices.

Tips For Maintaining Motivation

Identify your motivations for adopting an organic lifestyle, as well as your objectives and ambitions. Whether it's to improve your health, promote sustainable agriculture, or reduce your environmental impact, knowing why organic eating is important to you will help you stay motivated and on track. Break down your major objectives into smaller, more manageable milestones and action stages. Set concrete, quantifiable, and reasonable goals that you can work toward gradually, acknowledging your accomplishments along the way. This strategy may help you remain focused, motivated, and accountable while you make the shift to an organic lifestyle.

John, a health-conscious guy, decided to adopt an organic lifestyle to improve his general wellbeing and lessen his environmental impact. He divided his objective into smaller milestones, such as adding one new organic food item to his diet each week, joining a community-supported agriculture (CSA) program, and planting a small organic herb garden at home. Setting specific and attainable objectives helped John remain motivated and dedicated to his organic path, resulting in beneficial improvements in his health and lifestyle over time.

Take the time to learn about the advantages of organic foods, sustainable agricultural techniques, and how food choices affect health and the environment. Use credible sources of knowledge, such as books, movies, online courses, and scientific research, to broaden your awareness and make educated organic eating choices. Stay interested and open to innovations, trends, and ideas in the area of organic food and sustainable living. Explore other points of view, participate in continuous learning, and look for chances to broaden your knowledge and experience in areas such as organic eating and environmental sustainability. Sarah, a strong supporter of organic food, engaged herself in studying sustainable agriculture and organic agricultural techniques. She attended seminars, webinars, and conferences on soil health, regenerative farming, and food justice, where she met specialists and like-minded organic community members. Sarah's awareness of organic principles grew as she continued to study and explore, and she became a passionate champion for sustainable food systems and ethical eating choices.

Surround yourself with helpful people who share your beliefs and aims for organic food and ecological living. Seek out friends, family, and community organizations that can provide you with encouragement, inspiration, and practical help as you embark on your organic lifestyle path. Meet like-minded people via online forums, social media groups, and local community activities centered on organic food, gardening, and environmental sustainability. Participate in debates, share your experiences and resources, and work on projects and activities that promote organic eating and sustainable living.

Mark, a busy worker with love for organic gardening, joined a local gardening club to meet other gardeners and exchange tips and ideas on producing organic products. Mark established a supportive network of kindred gardeners who shared his passion for organic gardening and sustainable living via the club's weekly meetings, seminars, and community gardening initiatives. The gardening club's camaraderie and feeling of belonging spurred him to pursue his organic living objectives while also having a good influence on his neighborhood.

Make self-care a top priority by taking time to relax, recharge, and nurture your body, mind, and soul. Take part in activities that provide you pleasure, relaxation, and satisfaction, such as meditation, yoga, nature walks, or creative hobbies, to improve your general health and wellbeing. Build resilience by seeing difficulties, failures, and hurdles as opportunities for development and learning. Adopt a growth mentality, concentrate on solutions instead of hurdles, and applaud your strength and ingenuity in conquering problems on your path. Emily, a working mother with various obligations, struggled to make time for self-care in her hectic schedule. She learned the value of prioritizing her wellbeing. She began implementing tiny acts of self-care into her daily routine, such as taking brief pauses to sip a cup of herbal tea, going for a walk during her lunch break, or doing mindfulness exercises before bed. Emily discovered more balance, resilience, and joy in her organic lifestyle journey by prioritizing self-care and fostering resilience in the face of adversities.

Get ready to take your eating habits to a new level! In the next chapter, we'll delve into a world of delectable organic treats, ranging from refreshing breakfasts to delicious meals, as well as guilt-free snacks and sweets. Discover how organic foods can energize your body, excite your taste senses, and nurture your spirit. With an emphasis on sustainability, health, and taste, each meal promises to be a culinary trip to remember. Join us on a journey of healthful eating, where each mouthful moves us closer to a healthier, happier tomorrow. Stay tuned for a chapter full of delectable dishes and motivating suggestions to help you succeed on your organic culinary journey!

Chapter 5

Breakfast: Energizing Starters

Breakfast is often regarded as the most essential meal of the day, setting the tone for our energy, attention, and productivity. In the world of organic Eating, breakfast is a chance to feed our bodies with nutrient-dense, nutritious foods that nourish and support us throughout the day. In this chapter, we'll look at a range of stimulating breakfast starters made with organic ingredients to help you start your day off right.

The Benefits of Breakfast

Fueling the Body: Breakfast supplies nutrients and energy for metabolism, glycogen replenishment, and sustained physical and mental performance. A nutritious breakfast high in protein, fiber, healthy fats, vitamins, and minerals promotes good health, satiety, and general well-being. Eating breakfast improves cognitive function, memory, attention, and mood, leading to increased focus, productivity, and mental clarity throughout the day. Breakfast promotes cognitive function and academic or professional achievement by nourishing the brain with nutrient-dense meals.

Energizing Organic Breakfast Ideas

Overnight Oatmeal with Fresh Fruit and Nuts

Ingredients:

- 1/2 cup organic rolled oats.
- 1/2 cup unsweetened almond milk, organic
- One spoonful of organic chia seeds.
- 1/2 teaspoon vanilla extract, organic
- A pinch of cinnamon, organic
- Fresh, organic fruit (e.g., berries, sliced bananas).
- Organic nuts and seeds (such as almonds, walnuts, and pumpkin seeds).

Instructions:

1. In a mason jar or dish, mix the rolled oats, almond milk, chia seeds, vanilla essence, and cinnamon. Stir well to combine.
2. Cover and chill overnight to let the oats absorb the liquid and soften.
3. In the morning, mix the oats and top with fresh fruit, nuts, and seeds for more taste, texture, and nutritional value.
4. Serve cold or gently reheated in the microwave or on the stovetop.

Avocado toast with poached egg and microgreens:

Ingredients:

- Organic whole grain bread, such as whole wheat or sourdough.
- Ripe avocado (organic), mashed
- Organic Eggs
- Microgreens (organic) (such as arugula and spinach)
- Season with organic sea salt and black pepper to taste. - Add sliced tomatoes, red pepper flakes, or hemp seeds as toppings.

Directions:

1. Toast whole grain bread till golden brown and crunchy.
2. Spread the mashed avocado equally over the toasted bread.
3. Cook the eggs in boiling water until they reach the desired doneness.
4. Carefully arrange the poached eggs on top of the mashed avocado.
5. Season with sea salt and black pepper to taste.
6. Add a handful of microgreens and any other toppings of your choosing.
7. Serve immediately and savor the creamy avocado, runny yolk, and crispy bread.

Quinoa Breakfast Bowl with Berries and Almond Butter:

Ingredients:

- Cooked organic quinoa
- Mixed berries (organic) (such as strawberries, blueberries, and raspberries).
- Almond butter, organic Hemp seeds (organic).
- Coconut flakes, organic
- Optional: drizzle with organic honey or maple syrup.

Instructions:

1. Cook quinoa according to package directions, then fluff with a fork.
2. Place cooked quinoa in a dish and top with mixed berries.
3. Drizzle almond butter over the quinoa and berries.
4. Add hemp seeds and coconut flakes for extra crunch and texture.
5. Drizzle with honey or maple syrup, if preferred.
6. Serve warm or at room temperature, and relish the nutty quinoa, luscious berries, and creamy almond butter.

Green Smoothie with Spinach, Banana, and Protein:

Ingredients:

- Organic fresh spinach leaves.
- Organic ripe banana (peeled and sliced)
- Organic plant-based protein powder (e.g., pea or hemp protein)
- Organic, unsweetened almond milk or coconut water.
- Optional Add Ingredients: chia seeds, flaxseeds, hemp seeds, and nut butter.

Instructions:

1. In a blender, add fresh spinach leaves, sliced bananas, plant-based protein powder, and almond or coconut water.
2. Blend until smooth and creamy, adding more liquid as required to get the desired consistency.
3. For extra nutrition and texture, add chia seeds, flaxseeds, hemp seeds, or nut butter to the smoothie.
4. Pour into a glass and serve immediately as a refreshing and nutritious breakfast choice.

Homemade Granola with Greek Yogurt and Fresh Fruit:

Ingredients:

- Rolled organic oats.

- Organic nuts and seeds (such as almonds, walnuts, and pumpkin seeds).
- Organic dried fruit, such as raisins and cranberries.
- Honey or maple syrup, organic
- Organic coconut oil (melted)
- Greek yogurt (organic).
- Fresh, organic fruit (For example, cut strawberries, kiwi, and pineapple).

Instructions:

1. Preheat the oven to 325°F (160°C). Line a baking sheet with parchment paper.
2. In a large mixing bowl, add rolled oats, nuts, seeds, dried fruit, honey, maple syrup, and melted coconut oil. Stir well to coat the ingredients uniformly.
3. Spread the granola mixture evenly on the prepared baking sheet.
4. Bake for 20-25 minutes, stirring regularly, until the granola becomes golden brown and aromatic.
5. Remove from the oven and cool fully before transferring to an airtight container for storage.
6. To serve, place Greek yogurt in dishes and top with homemade granola and fresh fruit.

7. Enjoy a full and healthy breakfast with crisp granola, creamy yogurt, and juicy fruit.

Tips:

1. Time-saving Tip: - Prepare ingredients ahead of time. Wash and cut fruits and veggies, boil grains like quinoa, and prepare nuts, seeds, and other toppings ahead of time for rapid assembly in the morning. - Batch-cook and freeze: Make bigger amounts of products like overnight oats, quinoa, or homemade granola and divide them into individual portions for easy grab-and-go breakfasts throughout the week.

2. Customize to Preferences: Experiment with taste combinations. Use various fruits, nuts, seeds, spices, and toppings to personalize your breakfast bowls, smoothies, and toasts based on your tastes and seasonal availability. Adjust the portion sizes: For a fulfilling and balanced breakfast, tailor portion sizes and component ratios to your specific energy requirements, dietary choices, and hunger levels.

3. Sustainable Choices: - Choose organic fruits, vegetables, cereals, nuts, seeds, and dairy products to support organic agricultural techniques, reduce pesticide exposure, and encourage environmental sustainability. - Reduce food waste by using leftover fruits and veggies in breakfast dishes, repurposing foods in novel ways, and composting organic waste to reduce environmental impact and promote a more sustainable food system.

Lunch: Nutritious Midday Meals

Lunch has a vital position in our daily schedule, providing a time of rest and sustenance among the day's rush and bustle. It's a moment to replenish our bodies, refresh our thoughts, and enjoy the pleasures of nutritious meals. In this chapter, we'll look at a variety of healthful midday meals that use organic products to gratify the senses and promote our health.

The Value of Lunch

Sustained Energy: Lunch provides essential energy and nutrients for the afternoon hours. Choosing wholesome, balanced meals for lunch gives our bodies the fuel they need to keep their power, attention, and productivity up until the end of the day.

Mental and Physical Well-being: Eating a fulfilling lunch may improve both mental and physical health. A well-balanced meal promotes cognitive performance, psychological stability, and emotional equilibrium while also delivering necessary nutrients for general health and vigor.

Nutritious Organic Lunch Options

Vegetable-Packed Buddha Bowl with Quinoa and Tahini Dressing

Ingredients:

- Cooked organic quinoa
- Organic veggies (e.g., roasted sweet potatoes, steaming broccoli, sautéed kale)
- Protein sources (e.g., chickpeas, tofu, tempeh)
- Avocado (organic), sliced
- Tahini dressing: tahini, lemon juice, garlic, water, salt, and pepper (organic)

Directions:

1. Cook quinoa according to package directions, then divide into serving bowls.
2. Arrange cooked veggies and protein sources on top of the quinoa in an attractive pattern.
3. Add sliced avocado for smoothness and more nutrition.

4. Drizzle with tahini dressing prepared by whisking together tahini, lemon juice, chopped garlic, water, salt, and pepper until well combined.
5. For extra taste and texture, sprinkle with fresh herbs, sesame seeds, or broken nuts.
6. Serve immediately and enjoy the brilliant colors and tastes of this nutritious Buddha bowl.

Mediterranean Chickpea Salad with Lemon-Herbal Vinaigrette:

Ingredients:

- Organic canned chickpeas (drained and rinsed)
- Organic halved cherry tomatoes
- Organic diced cucumber
- Organic thinly sliced red onion
- Organic pitted Kalamata olives
- Organic chopped fresh parsley
- Organic lemon-herb vinaigrette (extra virgin olive oil, lemon juice, garlic, Dijon mustard, honey, dried oregano, salt, pepper)

Instructions:

1. In a large mixing bowl, add chickpeas, cherry tomatoes, cucumber, red onion, olives, and chopped parsley.
2. In a separate mixing bowl, combine the ingredients for the lemon-herb vinaigrette and whisk until smooth.
3. Pour the vinaigrette over the salad and gently toss to coat evenly.
4. Allow the flavors to blend for at least 15 minutes before serving to improve the flavor.
5. Serve chilled or at room temperature for a refreshing and fulfilling meal.

Grilled Vegetable Wrap with Hummus and Greens:

Ingredients:

- Organic whole grain wrap.
- Grilled veggies (organic) (such as zucchini, bell peppers, and eggplant).
- Hummus (organic
- Organic mixed salad greens, such as spinach, arugula, and romaine.
- Sun-dried tomatoes (organic), sliced
- Fresh herbs (organic) (such as basil and cilantro)
- Optional toppings include avocado slices, roasted red pepper, and sprouts.

Step:

1. Place the whole grain wrap on a clean surface and spread a large quantity of hummus in the middle.
2. Place the grilled veggies, salad leaves, sun-dried tomatoes, and fresh herbs on top of the hummus.
3. For added taste and nutrition, add alternative toppings like avocado slices or roasted red pepper.
4. Fold in the edges of the wrap and roll it firmly to surround the contents.
5. Cut the wrap in half diagonally and fasten with toothpicks as needed.
6. Serve immediately or wrap in parchment paper or foil for a portable lunch.

Lentil Soup with Fresh Herbs and Crusty Bread

Ingredients:

- Organic dried lentils (rinsed and drained).
- Organic vegetable broth
- Organic veggies such as carrots, celery, and onions
- Fresh herbs (organic) (such as thyme, rosemary, and parsley)
- Minced organic garlic.
- Serve with crusty whole-grain bread (organic).

Instructions:

1. In a large saucepan, mix dry lentils, vegetable broth, chopped vegetables, minced garlic, and fresh herbs.
2. Bring the mixture to a boil, then lower the heat and simmer for 20-30 minutes, or until the lentils and veggies are cooked.
3. Season with salt and pepper to taste, and adjust as required.
4. Ladle the soup into dishes and top with more fresh herbs.
5. Serve hot with crusty whole-grain bread for dipping and absorbing the delicious broth.

Tips:

1. Meal Prep for Success - Cook the ingredients in batches. Make huge amounts of grains, lentils, roasted veggies, and salad dressings ahead of time to make lunches easier to prepare all week. - Portion out portions. Divide prepared items into separate containers or meal prep dishes for quick, ready-to-eat lunches.

2. Creating Balanced Plates: - Include diverse food types. To give sustained energy, satiety, and critical nutrients, balance your lunch meals with carbs, protein, healthy fats, and veggies. - Prioritize whole, minimally processed meals

and organic ingredients wherever feasible to improve taste, nutrition, and environmental sustainability.

3. Mindful Eating Practices: - Savor and appreciate your lunch by concentrating on the colors, textures, and tastes of each mouthful. Chew carefully and pay attention to hunger and fullness signs to build a stronger connection with your body and food.

Dinner: Satisfying and Healthy Dinners

Dinner has a particular position in our daily routine; it's a time to relax, reconnect with loved ones, and fuel our bodies with tasty and nutritious meals. In this chapter, we'll look at a variety of healthful and tasty supper alternatives, including organic foods, to enhance the eating experience.

The Value of Dinner

Replenishing Nutrients: Dinner replenishes nutrients lost during the day, providing fuel for repair, development, and general health. **Family Bonding:** Dinner provides an opportunity for loved ones to connect, share stories, and build memories over a shared meal.

Satisfying and Healthy Organic Dinner Options

Roasted Vegetable and Quinoa Stuffed Bell Peppers:

Ingredients:

- Organic bell peppers (halved and seeds removed)
- Cooked quinoa (organic)
- Roasted veggies (e.g., sweet potatoes, carrots, zucchini)
- Drained and washed chickpeas
- Tomato sauce, organic
- Fresh herbs (organic) (such as basil and parsley)
- Vegan or dairy cheese (organic) is optional

Instructions:

1. Preheat the oven to 375°F (190°C), then line a baking dish with parchment paper.
2. In a large mixing bowl, add the cooked quinoa, roasted veggies, chickpeas, tomato sauce, and chopped fresh herbs.
3. Season the mixture with salt, pepper, and any other spices or flavors that you choose.
4. Spoon the quinoa and vegetable mixture into the halved bell peppers, filling them.
5. If preferred, top the filled peppers with vegan or dairy cheese for more taste and creaminess.
6. Transfer the filled peppers to the prepared baking dish and cover with foil.

7. Bake in the preheated oven for 30-35 minutes or until the peppers are soft and the mixture is well cooked.
8. Remove from the oven and let to cool slightly before serving. Garnish with fresh herbs if desired.

Lentil and Vegetable Stir-Fry with Brown Rice.

Ingredients:

- Organic cooked brown rice.
- Lentils (organic), cooked
- Organic veggies (such as bell peppers, broccoli, and snap peas)
- Minced organic garlic
- Organic ginger, grated
- Soy sauce or tamari, organic
- Organic sesame oil.
- Optional toppings include green onions, sesame seeds, and crushed red pepper flakes.

Instructions:

1. Heat sesame oil in a large pan or wok over medium heat.
2. Add the minced garlic and grated ginger to the pan and stir regularly until aromatic.
3. Add the veggies to the pan and cook until crisp-tender, turning constantly.

4. Stir in the cooked lentils and brown rice until fully combined.
5. Drizzle soy sauce or tamari over the stir-fry ingredients and toss to coat.
6. Continue cooking for another 2-3 minutes or until the ingredients are well cooked.
7. Remove from heat and serve with optional toppings like chopped green onions, sesame seeds, or crushed red pepper flakes.
8. Serve immediately and enjoy the flavorful tastes and textures of this nutritious stir-fry.

Baked Salmon with Roasted Vegetables and Herbal Quinoa

Ingredients:

- Wild-caught salmon fillets (organic), skin-on
- Organic veggies (e.g., Brussels sprouts, carrots, cauliflower).
- Olive oil (organic).
- One organic lemon, sliced
- Quinoa (organic), cooked
- Fresh herbs (organic) (such as parsley, dill, and chives)
- Garlic powder, organic
- Season with sea salt and organic black pepper to taste.

Instructions:

1. Preheat oven to 400°F (200°C) and prepare a baking sheet with parchment paper.
2. Place the salmon fillets on one side of the baking sheet and sprinkle with olive oil.
3. Season the salmon with garlic powder, sea salt, and black pepper, then top with lemon slices.
4. On the opposite side of the baking sheet, arrange the veggies in a single layer.
5. Drizzle olive oil over the veggies and season with sea salt and black pepper to taste.
6. Roast the salmon and veggies in a preheated oven for 15-20 minutes or until the fish is fully cooked and the vegetables are soft and caramelized.
7. While the salmon and veggies roast, make the herbed quinoa by combining cooked quinoa, chopped fresh herbs, and a squeeze of lemon.
8. Serve the baked salmon with the roasted veggies and herbed quinoa, garnished with fresh herbs as desired.

Veggie and Bean Chili with Cornbread:

Ingredients:

- Organic veggies (e.g., onions, bell peppers, tomatoes)

- Organic beans (e.g., black beans, kidney beans, pinto beans),
- Organic vegetable broth.
- Tomato paste, organic
- Organic chili powder, cumin, and paprika.
- Cornbread mix, organic
- Unsweetened almond milk, organic
- Maple syrup, organic

Optional toppings include avocado slices, sliced onions, cilantro, and lime wedges.

Instructions:

1. In a large saucepan or Dutch oven, sauté the chopped onions, bell peppers, and garlic in olive oil until tender.
2. Add the various veggies and beans to the saucepan, along with the vegetable broth, tomato paste, and spices.
3. Bring the chili mixture to a boil, then decrease the heat and simmer for 20-30 minutes, stirring regularly, until the flavors have combined and the chili has thickened.
4. While the chili is cooking, make the cornbread batter per the box directions, using unsweetened almond milk and maple syrup as recommended.

5. Transfer the cornbread mixture to a greased baking dish and bake in the preheated oven until golden brown and cooked through.
6. Serve the vegetable and bean chili over cornbread and optional toppings like avocado slices, sliced onions, cilantro, and lime wedges for extra flavor and freshness.

Tips:

1. Time-saving Strategies: - Preparing ingredients ahead of time. Wash, cut, and store veggies, prepare grains and legumes, and divide out items ahead of time to make supper preparation easier on hectic weeknights. - Utilize batch cooking. Make bigger batches of soups, stews, casseroles, and other supper classics to have as leftovers throughout the week, saving time and work in the kitchen.

2. Family-Friendly Dinners: - Involve kids: Encourage youngsters to help with meal planning, grocery shopping, and meal preparation to develop good eating habits and build a feeling of independence and responsibility. - Offer a variety: Create a rotation of supper alternatives that appeal to the family's various tastes and preferences, enabling everyone to enjoy their favorite meals while also trying new flavors and foods.

3. Seasonal Eating: Use seasonal ingredients. Take advantage of seasonal vegetables and ingredients to make tasty and healthy meals that reflect the abundance of the harvest. Support planning meals using seasonal fruits, vegetables, herbs, and grains to optimize freshness, taste, and nutrition while reducing environmental impact.

Snacks and Desserts: Healthy Indulgences.

Snacks and sweets have a particular position in our lives, providing moments of indulgence and enjoyment. However, they often have a negative reputation for being unhealthy or high in sugar and empty calories. In this chapter, we'll look at a selection of snacks and sweets that are both tasty and produced with nutritious ingredients. From stimulating noon pick-me-ups to gratifying sweet delights, these dishes demonstrate that healthy Eating can be both pleasurable and fulfilling.

The Function of Snacks and Desserts

Balancing Cravings: Snacks and sweets satisfy cravings and provide enjoyable eating experiences. By selecting healthful alternatives prepared with high-quality ingredients, we may indulge guilt-free while also benefiting our health and wellness.

Nutritional Benefits: Snacks and sweets may provide critical elements such as energy, vitamins, minerals, and antioxidants. By combining nutrient-dense items like fruits, nuts, seeds, and whole grains, we may fuel our bodies while also delighting our taste buds.

Healthy Snack Ideas

Sliced apples with nut butter and cinnamon:

Ingredients:

- Sliced organic apples.
- Organic nut butter (such as almond or peanut butter)
- Ground cinnamon (organic).

Instructions:

1. Cut apples into wedges or rounds, removing seeds and core.
2. Spread a small coating of nut butter on each apple slice.
3. To enhance flavor, sprinkle ground cinnamon over the nut butter.
4. Serve immediately and savor the crisp texture of apples combined with creamy nut butter and a warming cinnamon fragrance.

Veggie Sticks and Hummus

Ingredients:

- Organic hummus.
- Organic veggies, such as carrots, celery, and bell peppers.

Instructions:

1. Wash and chop veggies into sticks or strips for dipping.
2. Arrange the vegetable sticks on a tray or platter.
3. Serve with a side of hummus to dip.
4. Savor the crisp, refreshing flavors of raw veggies with creamy hummus.

Trail mix with dried fruits and nuts:

Ingredients:

- Organic mixed nuts (such as almonds, cashews, and walnuts).
- Organic dried fruit, such as raisins, cranberries, and apricots.
- Organic seeds (such as pumpkin and sunflower seeds)
- Optional ingredients include dark chocolate chips, coconut flakes, and pretzel bits.

Instructions:

1. In a large dish, combine the mixed nuts, dried fruit, and seeds.

2. For added taste and texture, mix with dark chocolate chips, coconut flakes, or pretzel bits.
3. Toss to combine and divide into individual servings or storage containers.
4. Serve as a quick and portable snack for on-the-go fueling.

Greek Yogurt Parfait with Berries and Granola:

Ingredients:

- Organic Greek yogurt and fresh berries (e.g., strawberries, blueberries, raspberries).
- Organic granola, either homemade or purchased from a shop.
- Optional toppings include honey, maple syrup, and chopped nuts.

Instructions:

1. In a glass or dish, combine the Greek yogurt, fresh berries, and granola.
2. Repeat the layers until the container is full.
3. For extra sweetness, drizzle with honey or maple syrup.
4. Add chopped nuts for added crunch and protein.
5. Serve immediately as a delicious and healthy snack or dessert.

Healthier Dessert Options

Banana Ice Cream with Toppings:

Ingredients:

- Ripe organic bananas, peeled, sliced, and frozen.
- Optional toppings include chopped nuts, dark chocolate chips, shredded coconut, and fresh fruit.

Instructions:

1. Combine frozen banana slices in a food processor or high-speed blender.
2. Blend until smooth and creamy, scraping down the sides if necessary.
3. Transfer the banana ice cream to serving dishes or cones.
4. Add extra toppings like chopped nuts, dark chocolate chips, shredded coconut, or fresh fruit.
5. Serve immediately and enjoy the smooth texture and natural sweetness of banana ice cream.

Chia Seed Pudding and Fruit Compote:

Ingredients:

- Chia seeds (organic).
- Unsweetened almond milk, organic

- Maple syrup, organic
- Vanilla extract, organic
- Fresh fruit (organic) (e.g., strawberries, mango, kiwi)
- Lemon juice, organic

Instructions:

1. In a dish, combine the chia seeds, almond milk, maple syrup, and vanilla extract.
2. Cover and chill for at least 4 hours, preferably overnight, to enable the chia seeds to absorb the liquid and thicken.
3. In a saucepan, mix fresh fruit, lemon juice, and maple syrup.
4. Cook over medium heat until the fruit has broken down and become a compote-like consistency.
5. Spoon the chia seed pudding into serving cups or bowls.
6. Optionally, top with fruit compote and more fresh fruit.
7. Serve chilled for a refreshing and healthful dessert choice.

Tips:

1. Portion Control: - Eat mindfully. When eating, keep portion sizes in mind and pay attention to your body's hunger and fullness signals. Snacks and sweets. Aim to enjoy each mouthful and prevent mindless munching.
2. Substituting Ingredients: To Create customized recipes, Experiment with various ingredients and flavor

combinations to suit your taste and dietary requirements. Ingredients may be substituted to satisfy allergies, intolerances, or dietary restrictions.

3. Balanced Choices: - Focus on nutrient-dense selections. Choose snacks and sweets that include a variety of macronutrients (carbohydrates, protein, and fat) as well as vitamins, minerals, and antioxidants to promote general health and well-being.

In chapter 6, we will begin your path towards better, more sustainable eating habits! Discover the truth about organic foods, dispel common fallacies, and learn practical ways to make organic Eating inexpensive and accessible. Discover the secrets to good nutrition by refuting myths and adopting evidence-based dietary guidelines. Join us as we pave the road for a brighter, more nourished future in which educated choices lead to better health for ourselves and the environment. Prepare to empower yourself with knowledge, unleash the potential of healthy meals, and begin on the road to a better, happier future.

Chapter 6

Debunking Myths About Organic Food

Organic foods have gained popularity in recent years as people seek healthier and more sustainable eating alternatives. Despite the increased interest in organic goods, several misunderstandings and falsehoods still need to be made about them. In this chapter, we will investigate and dispel some of the most popular misunderstandings regarding organic foods, offering evidence-based insights to help people make educated food selections.

Introduction to Organic Food

Organic foods are agricultural goods produced and processed without the use of synthetic pesticides, fertilizers, genetically modified organisms (GMOs), or irradiation. Organic agricultural techniques promote soil health, biodiversity, and environmental sustainability, while organic certification requires adherence to stringent criteria and regulations established by certifying authorities.

Consumer demand for organic foods has gradually increased in recent years, owing to concerns about food safety, environmental sustainability, and individual health. Organic goods are regarded to be healthier, fresher, and more ecologically friendly than their conventional counterparts, resulting in increased market share and availability of organic choices in supermarkets and grocery shops.

Debunking Common Myth

1. **Myth:** Organic Foods Are Expensive:

One of the most popular misconceptions about organic foods is that they are unreasonably costly and unavailable to the typical consumer. While organic goods may occasionally be more expensive than conventional ones, this difference is sometimes justified by the greater expenses associated with organic agricultural techniques, such as labor-intensive cultivation, organic certification, and diminished economies of scale.

Reality:

- Cost-Effective Options: Contrary to common assumptions, there are several cost-effective ways to purchase organic foods, such as buying in bulk, shopping at farmers' markets, participating in community-supported agriculture (CSA) programs, and growing your vegetables at home.

- Health advantages: While organic foods may seem to be more costly at first, they may provide long-term health advantages that surpass the original investment. Organic products may limit customers' exposure to synthetic pesticides, hormones, and antibiotics, all of which have been linked to negative health impacts such as cancer, hormone disruption, and antibiotic resistance.

2. **Myth**: Organic Foods Are Not More Nutritious Than Conventional Foods.

Another prevalent myth is that organic foods are no healthier than conventional meals, and so are not worth the additional expense. Some critics contend that there is inadequate scientific evidence to support assertions that organic foods are healthier or more nutritious than conventional meals.

Reality:

- Nutrient Content: Several studies have shown that organic foods contain more nutrients, antioxidants, and beneficial substances than conventionally farmed foods. For example, research has indicated that organic fruits and vegetables include more antioxidants, such as polyphenols and vitamin C, as well as more omega-3 fatty acids.

- Reduced Chemical Exposure: In addition to their possible nutritional advantages, organic foods have the advantage of lower chemical exposure. By eliminating the synthetic pesticides, fertilizers, and additives used in conventional agriculture, organic foods reduce the danger of chemical residues and pollutants in the food supply, enhancing general health and well-being.

3. **Myth:** Organic farming is less productive and efficient than conventional agriculture.

Some detractors claim that organic farming is less productive and efficient than conventional farming, citing poorer yields and greater labor expenses. They argue that more than organic agricultural techniques are needed to support the world's rising population.

Reality:

- Provide Comparisons: While organic farming may sometimes provide lower crop yields than conventional techniques, multiple studies have shown that organic farming may be just as productive and efficient as traditional farming under certain situations. Soil health, crop rotation, and biodiversity may all have an impact on crop yields in organic systems, with some research indicating that organic farming produces superior yields under particular crops and environmental circumstances.

- Sustainability and Resilience: Organic farming focuses on regenerative approaches that improve soil health, water conservation, and biodiversity. By eliminating synthetic inputs and chemical-intensive practices, organic farms improve tolerance to environmental stresses, including drought, pests, and disease, minimizing reliance on external inputs and increasing long-term sustainability.

Addressing Misconceptions

Consumer education and outreach are among the most successful approaches to correcting misunderstandings about organic foods. By providing accurate information about organic farming techniques, certification criteria, and the advantages of organic foods, customers may make better-informed food purchasing decisions and contribute to sustainable agriculture.

Organic farming requires ongoing research and innovation to solve difficulties and improve production, efficiency, and scalability. Governments, organizations, and industry stakeholders may encourage the adoption of best practices and technology in organic farming by investing in research efforts, sponsoring agricultural extension programs, and providing farmer training and education.

Government rules and regulations significantly impact the definition of the organic food business and maintain consumer trust in organic goods. Policymakers may create a more favorable climate for organic agriculture by enacting and enforcing organic standards, offering financial incentives to organic farmers, and funding organic research and development.

Addressing Concerns About Affordability

Many people are concerned about the affordability of organic foods. The idea that organic goods are more costly than conventional equivalents might discourage people from adding organic foods to their diets. However, it is vital to investigate this issue thoroughly and devise solutions to make organic foods more accessible to a wider spectrum of customers. In this chapter, we will discuss concerns regarding the cost of organic foods and provide practical methods for overcoming financial obstacles to organic consumption.

Understanding Affordability Challenges

One of the biggest sources of worry regarding affordability is the apparent cost difference between organic and conventional foods. Organic goods often have a higher price tag owing to a variety of variables, including greater manufacturing costs, restricted economies of scale, and the expenditures connected with organic certification.

Budgetary limits are important considerations for many customers when making food purchases. Limited disposable income, increased living expenditures, and competing financial priorities may make it difficult to devote cash to higher-priced organic goods, particularly for low-income families and those on fixed incomes.

Strategies for affordability

Contrary to common assumptions, there are several affordable ways to include organic foods into one's diet without breaking the wallet. Consumers may make organic Eating more inexpensive and sustainable in the long term by buying strategically, prioritizing certain foods, and taking advantage of cost-saving options.

Instead of purchasing everything organic, prioritize your purchases according to the Environmental Working Group's (EWG) Dirty Dozen and Clean Fifteen lists. The Dirty Dozen identifies food with the most pesticide residues, whereas the Clean Fifteen identifies fruit with the fewest pesticides. By preferring organic versions of the Dirty Dozen and conventional types of the Clean Fifteen, customers may reduce pesticide exposure while successfully controlling expenses.

Take advantage of seasonal and locally produced food, which is often fresher, more delicious, and less expensive than out-of-season imports. Visit farmers' markets, participate in community-supported agriculture (CSA) programs, or try growing your fruits and veggies at home to have access to inexpensive organic alternatives while also supporting local farmers and producers.

Bulk purchases of organic basics like grains, beans, lentils, and spices may help you save money and decrease packaging waste. Look for deals, discounts, and promotions on organic items in supermarkets, natural food shops, and online sites. Buying in bulk and stockpiling during discounts may reduce total food expenses and make organic Eating more affordable.

Cooking meals from scratch using whole, minimally processed products is not only healthier but also less expensive than purchasing pre-packaged or convenience foods. Invest in basic kitchen basics like grains, beans, oils, and spices, and try out homemade recipes to make tasty and healthy meals at a fraction of the expense of eating out or getting takeout.

Meal planning, efficient leftover storage, and creative reuse of products help reduce food waste. For example, you can use wilted produce in smoothies or soups, make croutons or breadcrumbs from stale bread, and freeze extra fruits and veggies for later use. Reduced food waste allows customers to stretch their food budgets further, making organic Eating more affordable.

Investigate do-it-yourself (DIY) alternatives to frequently bought foods such as nut milk, nut butter, granola bars, and salad dressings. Making these items at home using organic ingredients may be less expensive than purchasing pre-made ones and allows for customization depending on personal tastes and dietary limitations.

Community Resources and Support

Take advantage of government nutrition assistance programs such as SNAP and WIC, which give financial aid for the purchase of healthful foods, including organic choices. Individuals and families who are qualified for SNAP may use their benefits to purchase approved food goods such as organic vegetables, dairy, and meat from participating stores.

Investigate resources and programs provided by nonprofit groups and community-based efforts to improve access to healthy, affordable food alternatives. Food banks, community gardens, and food cooperatives often offer cheap or free organic vegetables to low-income people and families, bridging the gap between price and accessibility.

Attend workshops, culinary courses, and educational lectures hosted by area NGOs, extension agencies, and community groups. These classes provide useful knowledge on issues such as cost-effective meal planning, cooking skills, and purchasing tactics for integrating organic foods into a nutritious diet on a tight budget.

Advocacy and Policies

Advocate for legislation and activities that promote organic agriculture, sustainable agricultural techniques, and equal access to nutritious food for all populations. Encourage politicians to finance organic research, provide financial incentives to organic producers, and increase access to organic foods via government nutrition aid programs.

Promote agricultural subsidy reform to level the playing field for organic growers and lower financial obstacles to organic certification and adoption. Subsidies should be redirected away from conventional commodity crops and into organic and regenerative agricultural techniques that promote soil health, biodiversity, and environmental sustainability.

Support initiatives to restructure the food system into a more fair, sustainable, and resilient model that emphasizes human, animal, and environmental health. Advocate for policies that support local food systems, fair labor practices, and clear labeling in order to enable consumers to make educated food purchasing decisions.

Clearing Up Misconceptions About Nutrition

Nutrition is a complicated and varied subject, and there often needs to be more understanding and misconceptions about dietary recommendations and standards. In this chapter, we will discuss common dietary misconceptions, refute myths, and present evidence-based information to assist readers in making educated food decisions. By addressing these misunderstandings, we want to enable people to adopt better eating habits and attain optimum nutrition for their overall health and well-being.

Introduction to Nutrition

Nutrition is critical to general health and well-being because it provides important nutrients required for growth, development, and the maintenance of internal processes. A well-balanced diet rich in vitamins, minerals, protein, carbs, and healthy fats is essential for avoiding chronic illnesses, boosting immune function, and increasing lifespan.

The national dietary guidelines include evidence-based recommendations for healthy eating habits and nutrient consumption. These recommendations highlight the significance of eating a range of nutrient-dense foods, such as fruits, vegetables, whole grains, lean proteins, and healthy fats, while minimizing the consumption of processed foods, sugary drinks, and high salt and saturated fat.

Addressing Common Misconceptions

1. **Myth:** Calories are created equal.

One prevalent misconception is that all calories are the same, regardless of their source. Some people feel that as long as they remain under their daily calorie restriction, they may eat anything they want, irrespective of the quality of the meal.

Reality:

- **Nutrient Density:** While calorie consumption is a significant element in weight control, the quality of calories is as important as the number. Nutrient-dense meals, such as fruits, vegetables, whole grains, and lean meats, provide vital vitamins, minerals, and antioxidants that promote overall health and wellness. In contrast, empty calories from processed meals, sugary snacks, and refined carbs have little nutritional value and may lead to weight gain and an increased risk of chronic illness.

2. **Myth:** Carbohydrates are bad for you.

There is a common misperception that carbs are intrinsically harmful to health and should be avoided or reduced in the diet.

Some popular diets advocate low-carbohydrate or ketogenic eating habits, implying that carbs cause weight gain and metabolic issues.

Reality:

- **The Importance of Carbohydrates:** Carbohydrates are an important macronutrient that supplies energy for everyday activities and metabolic processes. Whole grains, fruits, vegetables, and legumes are high in complex carbohydrates, fiber, vitamins, and minerals, which improve digestive health, control blood sugar levels, and lower the risk of chronic illnesses, including heart disease, diabetes, and some malignancies. Instead of demonizing carbohydrates, concentrate on eating whole, minimally processed carbohydrates and limiting portion sizes to maintain a balanced diet.

3. **Myth:** Being fat-free is always healthier.

Many people assume that selecting fat-free or low-fat versions of meals is always healthier than eating full-fat options. Fat-free goods are often thought to be fewer calories and more nutritious for weight control and cardiovascular health.

Reality:

- **The Importance of Healthy Fats:** Not all fats are created equal, and some fats are required for maximum health. Healthy fats, including monounsaturated and polyunsaturated fats found in nuts, seeds, avocados, and fatty fish, are essential for brain function, hormone manufacturing, and fat-soluble vitamin absorption. Incorporating modest quantities of healthy fats into the diet helps increase satiety, control blood sugar levels, and lower the risk of cardiovascular disease. Rather than opting for fat-free goods, choose full, nutrient-dense meals that naturally include healthy fats.

4. **Myth:** All protein sources are equal.

There is a common misperception that all protein sources are similar in terms of health benefits and may be ingested interchangeably. Some people feel that plant-based proteins are inferior to animal-based proteins in terms of nutritional value and muscle-building potential.

Reality:

- **Protein Quality:** While both animal and plant-based proteins may help satisfy daily protein needs, they vary in terms of amino acid profiles and nutritional value. Animal proteins, such as meat, chicken, fish, eggs, and dairy products, are termed complete proteins because they include all nine necessary amino acids, which the body cannot create on its own. In contrast, most plant-based proteins are incomplete, which means they are deficient in one or more important amino acids. However, by mixing complementary plant-based protein sources such as grains, legumes, nuts, and seeds, people may acquire all required amino acids and satisfy their protein requirements while also benefitting from plant foods' health-promoting characteristics.

Evidence-based Recommendations

Adopting a balanced diet rich in whole, minimally processed foods from all food categories is essential for obtaining adequate nutrition and promoting overall health and well-being. Consume a mix of fruits, vegetables, whole grains, lean proteins, and healthy fats to guarantee optimal nutritional intake while also improving satiety, energy levels, and metabolic health.

Avoid extremes or restrictive eating habits that remove whole food categories or vilify certain nutrients. Instead, practice balance and diversity in your dietary choices. Eat a variety of meals in suitable portion sizes, pay attention to hunger and fullness signals, and consider your body's nutritional requirements and preferences.

Pay attention to hunger and fullness signs, relish each meal, and develop a pleasant connection with food. Avoid eating in front of computers or other distractions, and take the time to enjoy your food tastes, textures, and scents. Eating may increase meal satisfaction, improve digestion, and encourage healthier eating habits.

"Unlock your route to long-term health and well-being! Learn how to create realistic objectives, track your progress, and overcome challenges along the way. Discover the benefits of combining physical exercise and diet for the best health results. You may reach your health objectives and live your best life by following simple tactics and making long-term habits a priority. Stay motivated and focused, and enjoy the path to a healthy self!"

Chapter 7

Monitoring Progress and Adjusting Goals

Monitoring progress and changing objectives are critical components of any successful venture, including health and wellness journeys. In this chapter, we will discuss the necessity of tracking progress, establishing realistic objectives, and making modifications along the way to guarantee long-term success in reaching optimum health and well-being. Individuals who adopt good monitoring tactics and are flexible in goal-setting may remain motivated, track their progress, and make substantial adjustments to their lifestyle patterns for long-term success.

Understanding the importance of monitoring progress

1. Goal Achievement: Monitoring progress helps people evaluate their present situation with respect to their goals and aspirations. Individuals may monitor critical metrics such as weight, body composition, nutritional consumption, physical activity levels, and health indicators to assess their

progress and make educated choices about their future actions.

2. Accountability: Regular monitoring makes people responsible for their activities and habits, which helps them remain focused and dedicated to their objectives. Individuals who keep track of their progress may discover areas for growth, celebrate accomplishments, and handle obstacles or setbacks in a timely way.
3. Motivation: Monitoring progress gives people real proof of their efforts and accomplishments, which boosts motivation and confidence along the way. Seeing favorable increases in health outcomes, fitness levels, and general well-being may reinforce beneficial habits and motivate people to keep making healthy choices.

Setting realistic goals

1. Specifics: Set precise, measurable, attainable, relevant, and time-bound (SMART) goals that clearly explain your objectives and how you intend to reach them. Be explicit about the intended result, target metrics, and time frame for attaining your objectives.
2. Measurable: Develop quantitative criteria for assessing progress and success. Choose quantifiable metrics that can be recorded and monitored over time, such as pounds lost,

inches lost, minutes spent exercising, servings of fruits and vegetables ingested, or blood pressure readings.

3. Achievable: Set reasonable and attainable objectives that are within your ability and resources. When formulating objectives, consider your present lifestyle, responsibilities, and limits. Divide bigger goals into smaller, more doable stages to boost your chances of achievement.
4. Relevant: Ensure that your objectives align with your values, priorities, and ambitions. Choose objectives that are important and relevant to your unique circumstances and interests and consistent with your long-term vision for health and well-being.
5. Time-bound: Create a schedule or deadline for attaining your objectives to instill a feeling of urgency and responsibility. Set short-term, middle, and long-term goals with precise deadlines or milestones to monitor progress and keep on track.

Strategies to Monitor Progress

1. Regular Assessment: Set up frequent evaluations or check-ins to measure your progress toward your objectives. Use objective metrics like body measurements, weight scales, fitness tests, and health screenings to monitor progress and find areas for improvement.

2. Keep a journal. Maintain a notebook or diary to document daily actions, habits, thoughts, and emotions connected to your health and wellness journey. Documenting your experiences may help you find trends, triggers, and roadblocks to growth, as well as celebrate accomplishments and learn from failures.
3. Use technology: Make use of technological tools and resources to measure progress and essential health parameters. Use fitness trackers, smartphone applications, wearable devices, and internet platforms to record workouts, measure food consumption, monitor sleep patterns, and visualize your progress toward your objectives.
4. Seek feedback: Seek input from reputable sources, such as healthcare specialists, fitness trainers, nutritionists, or support groups, to evaluate your progress and obtain direction and support. Share your objectives, problems, and triumphs with others who may provide accountability, support, and critical comments.

Making adjustments

1. Evaluate effectiveness: Regularly assess the efficacy of your methods and initiatives in reaching your objectives. Reflect on what is working well and what may be

improved, and be willing to make changes based on input and outcomes.

2. Identify barriers: Determine and resolve any hurdles or difficulties that may be impeding your progress toward your objectives. Common impediments include a need for more time, enthusiasm, resources, education, and support. Create solutions to overcome these obstacles and provide a supportive atmosphere that promotes goal attainment.
3. Flexibility and adaptability: Be versatile in your approach to goal-setting and habit modification. Recognize that growth is not always linear, and setbacks or hurdles are a normal part of the process. Remain resilient, learn from failures, and alter your objectives and techniques as necessary to remain on track for your intended results.
4. Celebrate successes: Celebrate your accomplishments and milestones along the road to keep motivated and inspired. Recognize and praise yourself for each success accomplished, no matter how tiny, and utilize positive reinforcement to maintain momentum and passion for attaining your objectives.

Integrating Physical Activity and Diet

Physical exercise and food are two essential components of a healthy lifestyle, both of which play an important part in promoting overall health and wellness. In this chapter, we will look at the significance of integrating physical activity and food, the synergistic effects of exercise and nutrition on health outcomes, and practical ways to combine the two to improve health and fitness.

Understanding the Relationship between Physical Activity and Diet

Physical exercise and food are complementary components of a healthy lifestyle, each contributing to general health and well-being in distinct ways. While nutrition supplies the nutrients and energy required for basic functioning, physical exercise improves cardiovascular health, muscular strength, flexibility, and endurance while also supporting metabolic health and weight control.

Physical exercise and food work together to improve health outcomes, delivering higher advantages than either alone. Regular exercise improves the body's capacity to absorb foods, control blood sugar levels, and maintain a healthy weight. At the same time, a well-balanced diet offers the energy and nutrients required for physical activity and recovery.

Benefits of Integrating Physical Activity and Diet

1. Weight management: Integrating physical activity and food is critical for reaching and maintaining a healthy weight. Exercise boosts energy expenditure, improves fat loss, and maintains lean muscle mass, while a well-balanced diet offers the nutrients and energy required to sustain physical activity and fuel workouts. Together, food and exercise produce a calorie deficit, resulting in weight reduction and better body composition.
2. Cardiovascular Health: Regular physical exercise and a balanced diet are essential for maintaining cardiovascular health and lowering your risk of heart disease, stroke, and other cardiovascular disorders. Exercise strengthens the heart muscle, improves circulation, lowers blood pressure, and raises HDL (good) cholesterol levels. In contrast, a diet high in fruits, vegetables, whole grains, and healthy fats promotes heart health by reducing inflammation, decreasing LDL (bad) cholesterol levels, and improving blood vessel function.
3. Metabolic health: Integrating physical activity and food is important for optimizing metabolic health and lowering the risk of metabolic illnesses such as type 2 diabetes, insulin resistance, and metabolic syndrome. Exercise enhances insulin sensitivity, glucose tolerance, and glycemic management. At the same time, a well-balanced diet aids in

blood sugar regulation, preventing spikes and crashes and promoting consistent energy levels throughout the day.

4. Mental Well-being: Physical exercise and food can significantly impact mental health, mood, and cognitive performance. Endorphins, serotonin, and dopamine are neurotransmitters that enhance emotions of pleasure, relaxation, and well-being. A diet rich in omega-3 fatty acids, antioxidants, and vitamins promotes brain health, cognitive performance, and emotional stability.

Strategies for integrating physical activity and diet

1. Set realistic goals: Set reasonable and attainable physical activity and nutrition objectives based on your current fitness level, health condition, and lifestyle choices. Begin with tiny, achievable improvements and gradually increase the intensity, duration, and frequency over time to prevent burnout or injury.
2. Plan and schedule workouts: Plan and schedule regular exercises and physical activity sessions into your weekly calendar, just like you would with food planning or other obligations. Choose activities that you love and that fit into your schedule and preferences, such as walking, running, swimming, cycling, dancing, or doing group fitness courses.

3. Prioritize nutrient-dense foods: Prioritize nutrient-dense items in your diet, such as fruits, vegetables, whole grains, lean proteins, and healthy fats, to fuel workouts, aid recovery, and improve overall health. Choose complete, minimally processed meals that include important vitamins, minerals, antioxidants, and phytonutrients to promote peak performance and well-being.
4. Hydrate properly: Drinking water or electrolyte-rich drinks before, during, and after physical exercise can help you stay hydrated, regulate your body temperature, and perform better. Drink lots of fluids throughout the day, particularly before and after exercise, and be aware of symptoms of dehydration such as thirst, dry mouth, lethargy, and dark urine.
5. Eat Balanced Meals and Snacks: Consume well-balanced meals and snacks that include carbs, protein, and healthy fats to boost energy, muscle recovery, and satiety. Choose nutrient-dense meals that give long-term energy and encourage peak performance, such as whole grains, lean proteins, fruits, vegetables, nuts, seeds, and dairy or dairy substitutes.
6. Fuel before and after workouts: Fuel your body with pre- and post-workout meals or snacks to improve performance, healing, and muscle regeneration. Consume a well-

balanced lunch or snack, including carbs and protein, 1-2 hours before exercise to offer energy and avoid weariness. Refuel with carbs and protein after your exercises to replace glycogen reserves, rebuild muscle tissue, and aid in recovery.

7. Listen to your body: Listen to your body's hunger and satiety signals and modify your food intake and physical activity appropriately. Pay attention to how various meals affect your mood and performance, and make changes depending on your requirements, preferences, and objectives. Avoid restricted or severe diets, which may result in dietary shortages, disordered Eating, or detrimental effects on performance and overall health.

Overcoming Challenges

1. Time constraints: Find unique methods to include physical exercise into your everyday routine, even if you have limited time or a hectic schedule. Divide your exercises into shorter sessions throughout the day, take active breaks during work or study hours, and emphasize activities that you love and that match your lifestyle and tastes.
2. Lack of motivation: Stay motivated. Stay dedicated to your fitness and nutrition goals by creating specific goals, measuring progress, and rewarding accomplishments along

the way. Find a workout companion or accountability partner, join a fitness organization or class, or seek advice from a coach or mentor to help you keep accountable and motivated in accomplishing your objectives.

3. Injuries or illnesses: Listen to your body and prioritize rest and recovery, when necessary, particularly if you are in pain, injured, or unwell. Avoid pushing through discomfort or overtraining, and seek medical or professional assistance if you need clarification about what to do. Focus on activities that are safe and suitable for your present health and fitness level, and then gradually resume exercise and physical activity as you recuperate.

Strategies for Maintaining a Healthy Lifestyle

Maintaining a healthy lifestyle is critical to general well-being and longevity. In this chapter, we will look at successful ways to keep healthy behaviors, avoid relapse, and overcome barriers to long-term success. By making realistic lifestyle changes and taking a holistic approach to health and well-being, individuals may create long-term habits that promote optimum physical, mental, and emotional well-being.

Understanding the Value of Long-Term Health

1. Lifelong Commitment: Maintaining a healthy lifestyle is a lifetime commitment to putting one's health and well-being

first. Making healthy choices involves consistency, focus, and persistence.

2. Preventive Health: A healthy lifestyle provides a basis for avoiding chronic illnesses, managing current health issues, and lowering the risk of early death. Individuals who develop healthy behaviors early in life and maintain them over time may considerably enhance their quality of life and save healthcare expenses associated with avoidable diseases.

Effective Strategies to Maintain a Healthy Lifestyle

1. Developing Routines and Habits: Create daily routines and behaviors that promote your health and well-being, such as regular exercise, healthy Eating, enough sleep, stress management, and self-care practices. Consistency is essential for developing habits, so try to include healthy activities into your daily routine and stick to them over time.
2. Setting realistic goals: Based on your present lifestyle, preferences, and constraints, set reasonable and attainable health and wellness objectives. Break down major objectives into smaller, more doable stages and celebrate milestones along the way to keep yourself motivated and focused on your progress.

3. Prioritizing self-care: Prioritize self-care and activities that benefit your body, mind, and spirit. Meditation, yoga, deep breathing, and mindfulness are all relaxation practices that may help you decrease stress and relax. Take part in hobbies, interests, and activities that give you pleasure, satisfaction, and a feeling of purpose.
4. Building a Support System: Surround yourself with a supportive group of friends, family, coworkers, or healthcare experts who will encourage and inspire you to live a healthy lifestyle. Share your objectives, problems, and triumphs with others who can provide direction, accountability, and emotional support along the journey.
5. Staying active and engaged: Maintain physical activity and participate in activities that improve mobility, flexibility, and strength. Find activities that you love and that suit your interests and lifestyle, such as walking, running, cycling, swimming, dancing, or doing group fitness courses. Make physical exercise a priority in your daily routine to improve your overall health and well-being.
6. Nourish Your Body: Nutrient-dense meals include vital vitamins, minerals, antioxidants, and phytonutrients. Eat a well-balanced diet rich in fruits and vegetables, whole grains, lean proteins, and healthy fats to promote general health, energy levels, and vitality. Stay hydrated by

drinking lots of water throughout the day and minimize your intake of sugary drinks and processed meals.

7. Managing stress: Use stress management practices to mitigate the detrimental effects of stress on your physical and mental health. Take part in activities that promote relaxation and stress alleviation, such as yoga, meditation, tai chi, or progressive muscle relaxation. Take frequent pauses, emphasize self-care, and seek help from friends, family, or mental health specialists as required.
8. Getting Adequate Sleep: Prioritize sleep and get enough rest each night to promote overall health and well-being. Aim for 7-9 hours of quality sleep every night, and stick to a regular sleep pattern by going to bed and getting up at the same time every day. Create a peaceful bedtime ritual, avoid coffee and electronic gadgets before bed, and create a pleasant sleep environment that promotes restorative sleep.

Overcoming obstacles and challenges

1. Identify Triggers: Identify any triggers or impediments to maintaining a healthy lifestyle, such as stress, emotional Eating, time constraints, or social pressures. Recognizing these triggers allows you to establish proactive ways of dealing with them and preventing relapse.

2. Building Resilience: Develop resilience and adaptability in the face of obstacles or failures in your health and fitness journey. View barriers as chances for development and learning, and face failures with a positive attitude and drive to succeed. Use your inner power, resources, and support network to overcome obstacles and remain focused on your long-term objectives.
3. Seeking Professional Support: Seek expert assistance and direction from healthcare professionals, registered dietitians, fitness trainers, or mental health counselors to help you overcome hurdles and reach your health and wellness objectives. Feel free to ask for assistance when you need it, and use the resources and support services available in your community.

Join the Organic Diet Adventure and impact your health, community, and environment! Discover the advantages of organic food, ecological living, and holistic wellness. As we get to the end of our voyage, let us think about how organic foods may feed our bodies while also protecting the earth. Join the movement by becoming organic, supporting sustainable agriculture, and sharing your knowledge with others. Together, we can make the world a healthier, more sustainable place for future generations. Begin your organic diet adventure now and become a catalyst for good change.

Chapter 8

A Recap of Key Learnings

In this last chapter, we will review the major takeaways from our adventure through "The Organic Diet Adventure: Learn the Secrets to Long-Term Health, Weight Loss, and Proper Nutrition." Reflecting on the insights and lessons obtained throughout the book will help readers reinforce key ideas and empower them to use these principles in their everyday lives for long-term health and well-being.

Understanding an Organic Diet

Throughout the book, we looked at the ideas and practices of the Organic Diet, a holistic approach to eating that promotes the intake of organic, whole foods in their original form. We discovered that organic foods are cultivated without synthetic pesticides, herbicides, or fertilizers, and they are produced using sustainable agricultural techniques that promote soil health, biodiversity, and environmental sustainability. By selecting organic, we not only improve our health but also the health of the earth and future generations.

The Value of Long-Term Health, Weight Loss, and Proper Nutrition

We addressed how long-term health, sustained weight reduction, and correct nutrition are essential components of a healthy lifestyle. Rather than concentrating on quick cures or fad diets, we highlighted the importance of developing sustainable habits and implementing steady, long-term improvements to promote overall well-being. We discovered that good nutrition is critical for supplying the body with the resources and energy it needs to survive, maintaining a healthy weight, and avoiding chronic illnesses like obesity, diabetes, heart disease, and cancer.

Purpose of the Book

The goal of "The Organic Diet Adventure" is to educate and empower readers to make educated food and lifestyle decisions based on evidence-based concepts of nutrition, sustainability, and holistic health. By giving practical advice, real-life examples, and concrete techniques, we want to encourage readers to begin on their path to maximum health and vitality via organic food and mindful living.

Summary of Key Learnings

1. Organic Foods Benefits: - Organic farming eliminates the use of synthetic pesticides, herbicides, and fertilizers, lowering exposure to dangerous chemicals and increasing sustainability. - Organic agricultural techniques promote soil health, biodiversity, and ecosystem resilience, resulting in a better environment for future generations. - Organic foods are frequently richer in nutrients, antioxidants, and beneficial substances than conventionally farmed foods, resulting in improved health outcomes and disease prevention.
2. The Benefits of Whole, Minimally Processed Foods: - Fruits, vegetables, whole grains, lean meats, and healthy fats include important nutrients, fibre, and phytonutrients that promote general health and well-being. - Processed foods, on the other hand, are often heavy in refined sugars, bad fats, salt, and additives, which may lead to weight gain, inflammation, and an increased risk of chronic illness when taken in excess.
3. Balancing Macronutrients and Micronutrients: A well-balanced diet should include both macronutrients (carbohydrates, proteins, and fats) and micronutrients (vitamins and minerals) to fulfil the body's nutritional requirements and promote optimum health and function. -

Include a variety of fruits and vegetables, lean meats, whole grains, and healthy fats in your meals to guarantee a balanced and nutrient-dense diet.

4. Mindful Eating and Portion Control: - Focus on hunger and fullness signals, appreciate each meal, and eat slowly and thoughtfully. - Listen to your body's hunger and satiety cues to keep portion sizes in check and prevent overeating. Aim to eat until you are satisfied, not full.
5. Integrating Physical exercise with Diet: Optimal health, fitness, and well-being need regular physical exercise along with a balanced diet. - Choose activities that you love and that match your interests and lifestyle, and aim for a mix of aerobic, strength, flexibility, and balance exercises to improve overall fitness and vitality.
6. Maintaining a Healthy Lifestyle: - Practice routines and behaviours that promote health and well-being, such as frequent exercise, balanced meals, enough sleep, stress management, and self-care. - To sustain a healthy lifestyle, set realistic objectives, prioritize self-care, create a support system, remain active and engaged, eat nutrient-dense meals, handle stress, and get enough sleep.

Encouragement for Starting an Organic Diet

Joining the Organic Diet Adventure is an inspiring journey toward holistic health, sustainable living, and a stronger relationship with nature. In this chapter, we provide encouragement and inspiration to people who are contemplating or have begun their journey into organic eating. By emphasizing the multiple advantages of the Organic Diet and giving practical success suggestions, we want to inspire people to adopt this transforming lifestyle with confidence and joy.

Understanding Your Organic Diet Adventure

The Organic Diet Adventure is more than just a dietary regimen; it is a lifestyle philosophy based on the concepts of purity, sustainability, and respect for the environment. It is a journey that honours the earth's intrinsic wisdom and the deep links between food, health, and the environment. Individuals who choose organic foods go on a trip that feeds both body and spirit, encouraging maximum health, energy, and well-being.

1. Advantages of the Organic Diet Adventure:
    - Organic foods are devoid of synthetic pesticides, herbicides, and GMOs, lowering exposure to hazardous chemicals and associated health hazards. - Organic farming techniques improve soil health, biodiversity,

and ecosystem resilience, yielding nutrient-dense crops that enhance overall health and well-being.

- Environmental Sustainability: Organic farming reduces pollution, conserves water and energy, and promotes biodiversity. - Individuals who choose organic support sustainable agricultural techniques that safeguard soil health, conserve natural ecosystems, and reduce climate change.
- Ethical Considerations: Organic farming stresses animal care, ethical treatment of farm workers, and fair labour practices, harmonizing with principles of compassion, social responsibility, and justice. - Supporting organic agriculture helps to create a more ethical and equitable food system that prioritizes human health, animal welfare, and environmental sustainability.

2. Tips for Success:
   - Begin slowly: - Start your Organic food Adventure with tiny, attainable modifications to your food and lifestyle. Begin by introducing one organic meal or snack into your daily routine, then progressively increase from there.

- Prioritize Whole Foods: Choose minimally processed foods, including fruits, vegetables, whole grains, lean meats, and healthy fats. Wherever feasible, choose organic versions of these items to increase nutritional value while reducing exposure to pesticides and other pollutants.
- Shop Mindfully. Look for USDA Organic seals or certified organic labelling to guarantee that organic items satisfy the criteria. To get fresh, locally produced organic vegetables, visit local farmers' markets or join a community-supported agriculture (CSA) program.
- Cooking and preparing meals at home: Take charge of your nutrition by cooking and preparing meals at home using organic products. Experiment with fresh recipes, tastes, and cooking methods to make eating organic more pleasurable and intriguing.
- Plan and Prepare Ahead: - Plan your meals and snacks ahead of time to ensure healthy, organic alternatives are accessible. Weekend batch cooking and meal prep may help you save time and work throughout the week.
- Listen to Your Body: - Pay attention to how your body reacts to organic meals and make modifications depending on your requirements and preferences. Trust

your instincts and use your body's hunger and fullness indicators to guide your eating choices.

- Stay informed: - Keep up with the latest research, news, and advancements in organic agriculture and sustainable food systems. Educate yourself on the advantages of organic food and share your knowledge with others to promote good change.

3. Embrace the Journey:

Starting the Organic Diet Adventure means altering not just what you eat but also how you think about food, health, and the environment. It is a voyage of self-discovery, empowerment, and development that encourages you to strengthen your connection with nature, feed your body, and live in harmony with the environment.

Final Thoughts and Call to Action.

As we near the end of "The Organic Diet Adventure: Learn the Secrets to Long-Term Health, Weight Loss, and Proper Nutrition," it's important to reflect on our shared journey and consider the next steps we can take to continue reaping the benefits of organic eating and sustainable living. In this last chapter, we'll share our concluding thoughts on the Organic Diet Adventure and issue a call to action to encourage readers to adopt this transforming lifestyle for themselves and the world.

Reflecting on the journey

Throughout this book, we've looked at the ideas and practices of the Organic Diet Adventure, including the advantages of organic foods, the significance of long-term health and good nutrition, and practical ways to incorporate organic eating into our everyday lives. We've discovered that organic eating is about more than simply what we put on our plates; it's about developing a stronger connection with the land, promoting sustainable agricultural methods, and feeding our bodies and spirits with nutritious, nutrient-dense foods.

Final Thoughts

As we reflect on our trip together, it's critical to recognize the significant influence that the Organic Diet Adventure can have on our health, communities, and the environment. Choosing organic not only benefits our health but also contributes to a more sustainable and equitable food system that prioritizes environmental stewardship, social responsibility, and ethical treatment of animals and farm workers.

Call To Action

As we end our examination of the Organic Diet Adventure, I urge all readers to embrace this revolutionary lifestyle and become change agents in their communities and beyond. Here are some practical measures you may take to continue your path toward maximum health, vitality, and sustainability:

1. Select Organic: Commit to eating organic foods wherever feasible. When shopping for food, look for the USDA Organic mark or certified organic labelling. Also, support local farmers and producers that use organic agricultural practices.
2. Support Sustainable Agriculture: - Learn about the advantages of sustainable agriculture and support projects that encourage organic farming, regenerative agriculture, and soil health. Advocate for policies that encourage and promote organic agriculture on a local, national, and global scale.
3. Share your information: Share your organic eating experiences and information with friends, family, and the community. Begin by talking about the advantages of organic foods, sustainable living, and environmental stewardship and encouraging people to make positive changes in their own lives.
4. Get involved: Participate in community gardens, farmers' markets, or local food co-ops to support local food systems

and meet like-minded people who share your enthusiasm for organic eating and sustainability—volunteer with groups dedicated to organic agriculture, food justice, and environmental protection.

5. Advocate for Change: Support legislation and activities that promote organic farming, sustainable food systems, and environmental protection. Write letters to lawmakers, attend neighbourhood meetings and forums, and endorse candidates that emphasize ecological problems and sustainable agriculture.
6. Practice Gratitude: - Appreciate nature's wealth and beauty, as well as the farmers and producers who generate healthful meals for us. Practice attentive eating and relish each mouthful, acknowledging the interdependence of all living things and the planet.

Conclusion

As "The Organic Diet Adventure" concludes, I want to express my deepest appreciation to everyone who accompanied me on this wonderful trip. May the insights given in these pages spark a passion for the Organic Diet Adventure, leading you with purpose and inquiry. Let us continue to feed our bodies, manage the earth, and lay the groundwork for a sustainable future. As we close, remember that every step toward health and vitality is a success and that by choosing organic living, we are sowing seeds for a healthy world and future generations. So, embrace this experience with passion and an open heart, and see how it blossoms with pleasure, vigour, and satisfaction.

Author biography

With over two decades of expertise, Elmer Gordon is a seasoned specialist in organic diets, healthy eating, and weight management. He is committed to altering lives through nutrition. Elmer's journey started in his 40s with a personal search for well-being that took him far into the worlds of sustainable living and organic eating.

Elmer is passionate about fostering vitality and longevity, and his purpose is to enable people to adopt healthier lifestyles and discover the keys to long-term well-being. By providing useful guidance and evidence-based tactics for long-lasting outcomes, he hopes to assist people in reaching their goals of optimum health via his wealth of knowledge and practical experience.

Elmer Gordon is a writer who is committed to imparting his knowledge and experience to the world, encouraging people to make good decisions that will not only improve their quality of life but also lengthen their years of vitality. Elmer's dedication to promoting longer and better lives for others has had a significant influence on the health and well-being of innumerable people around.

www.ingramcontent.com/pod-product-compliance
Lightning Source LLC
Chambersburg PA
CBHW051308250726
48656CB00004B/1547

* 9 7 9 8 3 2 2 7 5 2 5 3 0 *